About the Author

Louis Calvete was born in London of Spanish parents and grew up in a bilingual environment during the political, technical and stylistic events described in this book.

He spent the war years in Ecuador, South America and on returning to Britain, became in turn an industrial chemist, statistician, export manager, tour guide and translator.

Private sources of information have enabled him to reconstruct events which occurred during his childhood of which he was mostly unaware at the time and about which many are unaware today. His main interests are history, music and technology.

CW01019318

To Joanne
My favourite
daughter called
Joanne LoL
Louis

Publish and be damned
www.pabd.com

Permanent Waving

The Golden Years

by
Louis Calvete

Publish and be damned
www.pabd.com

First published in Canada 2006 by Louis Calvete.
The moral right of Louis Calvete to be identified as the author of this work has
been asserted.

louis@calvete.fsnet.co.uk

Designed in Toronto, Canada by Adlibbed ltd.
Printed and bound by Lightningsource in the US or the UK.

ISBN: 1-897312-34-2

Dedicated to the memory of Isidoro Calvete

(1886 - 1965)

and

G. James Calvete

(1910 - 2006)

Messrs. I. Calvete Ltd. have been producers of all kinds of electrical hairdressing equipment since 1917 and the designer of this system is a man who has been responsible for some of the most notable inventions in the Trade.
The Manual of the Permanent Waver - J. Bari-Woollss, 1934

To Eugene v.t., to have a permanent wave, e.g. "I must have my hair eugened for tonight"
English usage in the 1930s.

For whom are you carefully dressing your golden hair, simply but with such style?
Horace, Roman poet, 19 B.C.

The Swatch Store
104-106 Long Acre
Covent Garden
London
WC2E 9NR
Tel : 02078365663

RECEIPT / INVOICE

SFP108 (4) Bubblehop
    50.00 * 1   50.00

TOTAL (GBP)   50.00

CASH   50.00 GBP

VAT(4) 17.50%   7.45 GBP
TOTAL w/o VAT   42.55 GBP

Served by SEBASTIAN Number of items : 1
Ref.S_CG-2-35686 VPM 3
                        20/02/2007 12:19:17

AS_CG-0-42619

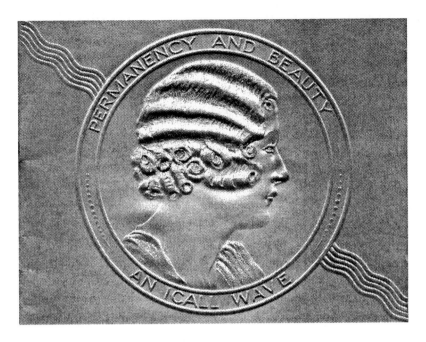

Centenaries of 1906

First attempt at electrical permanent waving of hair (Nessler)

Foundation of the London College of Fashion

The Hairdressers' Journal is 125 years old.

Approaching Centenaries of 1914 to 1939

The Modernist movement of design and the Art Deco form of art.

The first practical electrical permanent waving process (Eugene Suter – Isidoro Calvete)

The start and end of the First World War

[Above: From the silver cover of an Icall catalogue of 1934.]

Synopsis

In the 1920s and 30s, a period in which there emerged a movement of new types of design now called "Modernism", the name "Eugene" was a household name for a new technology and style of hairdressing called "electrical permanent waving" (or "perming") which was known to nearly every ladies' hairdresser and his clients. With the onset of war in 1939, this universally known method as then practised, lingered on until about 1950 and then totally disappeared so that it is virtually unknown today, although the knowledge acquired then lives on in modern salons.

In March, 2006 some newspapers (see Appendix II) decided unofficially to celebrate the notional centenary of the permanent-waving of hair. This was based on the fact that a German hairdresser, Karl Nessler, had invented in 1905 an electric "permanent-waving" machine which he demonstrated to the public on the 8th October 1906 in Oxford Street, London. The trade appears to have been indifferent to this event at the time, and it was not even reported in the Hairdressers' Journal. Of course, non-electric permanent-waving already existed before that, for example, as Marcel waving which used heated tongs. However, the first attempts by Nessler were so impractical and dangerous in the extreme that hairdressers continued to use the tried and trusted Marcel method. Nessler patented his process in 1909, but when the First Great War started, he fled England, where as a German he could be interned as an undesirable alien, and managed to get to the United States in 1915, where he continued his interest in the process.

This method of permanent waving really took hold when a Swiss national living in London, called Eugene Suter, saw the potential behind the idea - if its many drawbacks could be overcome, - and started trying to design his own equipment, while running his own hairdressing salons in the West End of London. However, Eugene (by which name he became universally known), like his predecessor Nessler was a competent hairdresser, but had no technical training. In 1917, in what was practically an accidental meeting, Eugene consulted my father, Isidoro Calvete, on the design of the most critical part of the equipment - the heaters. My father, who was a competent professional electrician, who had never dreamt of being involved in ladies' hairdressing, - but had started the manufacture of early electrical equipment for medical and beauty treatment, - redesigned the heaters, not knowing that for twenty years he would be involved in the forefront of permanent waving, a field in which he had had no previous experience, but which would make great strides because of the publicising ability of Eugene. By the 30's practically every woman in this country knew about "the Eugene process" and probably went to the hairdresser on a regular basis to have their hair re-permed as the hair grew out. If I had to choose a year on which to base the centenary, I would go for 1918, the year in which Eugene and my father combined the hairdressing skill and vision of one and the technical and commercial acumen of the other, to create equipment and styles which would dominate hairdressing.

Until 1930, an unusual situation existed in which I. Calvete Ltd manufactured all the equipment sold and used by Eugene, while at the same time selling similar equipment on its own account. Eugene was a great publicist and his name became synonymous with permanent-waving; on the other hand, I. Calvete Ltd led on the technical front and won more than its fair share of hairdressing competitions.

This unusual symbiosis lasted until 1930 with inevitable friction arising from intense mutual competition, and what had started as friendship gradually changed to antagonism, so that in the end Eugene withdrew from the arrangement and started manufacturing on his own account or found another manufacturer.

ii

However, with the depression and the threat of war Eugene eventually took over I. Calvete Ltd and the combined firm only lasted in its original form until shortly after the start of the Second World War.

Many of the names and equipment of this period mentioned in this book largely disappeared with the start of the Second World War, and the accomplishments of these pioneers seem to be have been largely forgotten, but many of the techniques, styles and technology have been assimilated into the wide variety of styles and methods that exists in the ladies' hairdressing world of today.

The developments mentioned in this book ran parallel with the technical and political events of that period. The year 1918 saw the end of the Great or First World War, a disastrous conflict which re-drew the map of Europe, made huge social changes and bankrupted the major powers. All this would have been worthwhile if, as had been hoped, this had resulted in a permanent peace. However, a series of uncontrolled international events took place, which not only had a dire effect on commerce and industry, but finally led to the Second World in 1939.

During this inter-war period, called by some the Modernist Period, daring advances took place in the Arts and Architecture which came to affect everyday life. From the social point of view, two other, highly relevant factors came into play.

The first, a social one, was the (partial) liberation of women. Although there was still a general feeling that the place of women (certainly married ones) was in the home, they were participating more and more, even before the First World War, in industry and other activities such as politics, and this was greatly emphasised during the war when there was a great shortage of male labour. Although recognition remained an uphill struggle, Oxford opened to women in 1920 and a level of enfranchisement was granted to women in 1918. And even if some restrictions still remained, this new freedom was reflected in major changes of dress and hair styles, which had a big effect on how women were perceived.

The other factor, a technological one, was the increasing availability of electricity and of electrical equipment for small businesses and domestic use. This was particularly marked in the case of the professional women's hairdresser who from having to deal with the old, conventional hairstyles responded to the demand for innovation and then led with new styles. This could hardly have been possible without the aid of the range of electrical equipment that was placed at their disposal and a greater understanding of the physics and chemistry of hair. Some of the wilder ideas may have disappeared, but many of the items used today, both professionally and in the home, derived one way or another from this period. Look in any ladies' hairdresser, Mail Order Catalogue or Electrical Goods Shop.

The main purpose of this book is to fill a gap in the history of hairdressing in the critical development of the profession between the wars. Apart from the initial dabbling by Nessler and the later publicity given to the styles of the eccentric Raymonde, important contributors to hairdressing such as Bari-Woollss, Eugene and Calvete remain unknown and unrecorded. The aim of this book is at least partially to correct this by giving an account of the creation and development of a business (I. Calvete Ltd) which was involved in the design and manufacture of equipment for use in ladies' hairdressing and beauty during the period 1917 to 1939, in the form of permanent-waving and, incidentally, medical equipment for the professional and beauty professions and home use, which were used at that time.

Most people form an image of history as a mental tapestry of major events. My feeling is that in an account such as this which consists of relatively minor events, the course these take are affected to a greater or lesser degree by the major ones which occur in the background. The inter-war period was one of intense economic and political upheaval, and these certainly affected the events which are related in this book, so I include a parallel mention of political and other events which took place at the same time and indirectly affected the course of contemporary affairs, including hairdressing.

Contents

Preface

In the year 2004, the Museum of London presented an exhibition called "1920s London". [18] My daughter Claire who is keen on history, art and fashion, particularly of that period, asked me to accompany her to the Exhibition, which I gladly did. After passing through various interesting sections, such as dresses, ballet, the 1924 Empire Exhibition and transport, we came to a section on machines and the use of electricity, which was just becoming available to the public in those years. Turning a corner, we came face-to-face with a seated, female mannequin bearing the suspended curlers of an old permanent-waving machine. The notice said "Hair-dressing equipment by Eugene Ltd, February 1923".

This immediately awoke memories of my childhood. During my first fifteen years, I lived in an environment in which conversations between my father and others often referred to the technical and financial implications of ladies hairdressing and permanent waving, often carried out in a mixture of English, Spanish and French (bigoudis, mise-en-plis, etc.) If a friend were to ask what my father did, it would be difficult to explain; all I knew, was it was something to do with electricity and women's hair - I sometimes wished he had been something easier to understand, such as a solicitor or a plumber. Claire said I should write a book on my father's contribution to hairdressing. Easily said, but I had been only a child during those years. However, after examining the materials at my disposal, I found that I had a fair number of

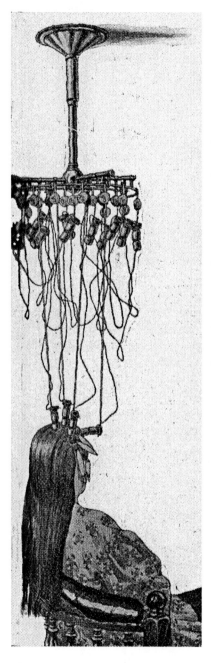

A 1920 permanent-waving machine sold by Eugene loosely based on the earlier Nessler model, but with improved heaters. The machine was fixed to the ceiling which meant moving the clients to the machine rather than the other way round, as was to be developed shortly afterwards by I. Calvete. The chandelier was also changed to the circular, mobile form which made it easier to use.

PREFACE

relevant photographs of the period, my father's diaries, and some catalogues[1].Unfortunately, my father died in 1965, but I had the memories of my brother who, being somewhat older than myself, had actively participated in many of the events of that time. In fact, when I showed him the post-card I had bought at the Museum of London, his reaction was "Goodness! That must be one of the earliest models that father made at Newman Street for Eugene!".

I imagine that by the 1930's something like this machine would be familiar to most women, from the simplest office worker to the richest society hostess if, as most urban women did, they regularly visited a hairdressing salon. However, production of equipment stopped during the Second World War, and afterwards, a change in styles and of technology meant that by the fifties these would largely have disappeared. Thus after some three generations, anyone shown such a machine on its own, would have difficulty in guessing its purpose. Seen in isolation, the impression is given of a science-fiction device for brain-washing!

Then, in May, 2006, another similar big exhibition took place, this time at the Victoria and Albert Museum in South Kensington, London. It was called : Modernism: Designing a new world, 1914-1939. This name has been applied to the period which corresponds almost exactly with that dealt with the period dealt with in this book. The exhibition had rather fewer artefacts than "20s London" but rather more of the philosophy of a new utopia. A healthier and happier new life was sought by designing better buildings, furniture and living conditions. "No new idea was more central to the dreams of a new utopia than that of technology, represented in word and image by "the machine". In addition, "Modernism was permeated by a deep concern for health[19] It was natural, therefore, that technology came to be applied to health, and hence to beauty.

I have noticed that the events recorded herein run parallel with the dramatic inter-war political events which acted as a sinister background to life at the time, even with something as innocent as

3

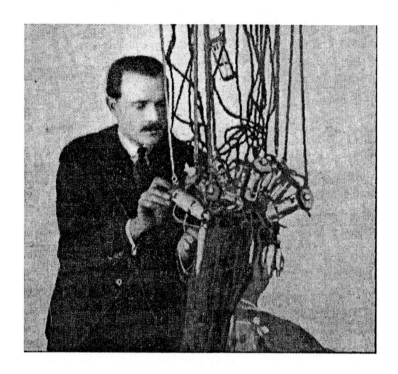

A 1920 photograph of "Mr. Eugene fitting the combined heaters over the curlers". This machine is the same type as shown on the previous page. The heaters were claimed to have "two divisions which render the different degrees of heat required by the roots and the ends of the hair" on the curler. This was part of an extensive advertising campaign by Eugene which seemed directed more at attracting clients to his hairdressing salon than to selling machines. At that time, he had premises at 23, Grafton Street, W.1. having moved there from 178, New Bond Street, W.1. In 1929, he moved to 31, Dover Street, Piccadilly, W.1, while by 1937 he was in 15/16 New Burlington Street.

4

PREFACE

hairdressing. They were to put an end to I. Calvete Ltd. as we knew it, and overwhelm our personal lives as well. So I include references to these events in italics, for those who, many years on, are unfamiliar with them, and they may be omitted if you are interested only in the hairdressing side of the story.

There is probably is a great deal that has been omitted from this narrative, but I have made some attempt at covering the multitude of different manufacturers and systems of permanent waving that arose in the inter-war years. There are other sources for such information and I shall quote some. However, my main object is to trace the rise and end of I. Calvete Ltd founded by my father, using the information readily to hand, with an unashamedly personal slant. At the same time, I have tried to give due credit to Eugene who, given his contribution to hairdressing, seems to have received little historical recognition. I apologise, if in this process I have inadvertently committed any errors or ruffled any feathers, or omitted any mention of copyright. At this distance in time it has not been possible to determine what has happened to the companies mentioned herein if indeed they still exist. So any existing trade-marks and copyright are readily acknowledged.

Throughout, Icall is the trade-name of I. Calvete Ltd and HJ stands for Hairdressers' Journal, now known as Hairdressers Journal International.

A background to permanent-waving

This book does not pretend to be a complete book on hairdressing or even of the history of hairdressing, but a few elementary facts will serve as a back-drop to the facts.

Hairdressing can be seen as a combination of two factors which inevitably overlap, but which, for convenience, I shall call "hygiene" and "style".

Starting with **_hygiene_**, the _comb_ is perhaps the earliest hairdressing tool and has been found in wide-spread archaeological sites of great antiquity. Being hand-made from natural materials such a bone or horn and difficult to make, it tended to be the possession of persons of status, and could be enhanced with engraving or precious metal. The purpose of a comb is to disentangle the hair and make it tidier. The process is analogous to the carding of wool, but before the availability of anything better, the wool was "teased" using the head of the teasel plant, thus preparing the wool for the spinning, and eventual weaving, processes. Given the antiquity of the use of wool for clothing, we do not know whether the combing or carding processes came first, or whether anything like teasel was used on human hair. The _brush_ can be considered as a kind of replacement of the comb, although it is not as efficient for disentangling the hair. However, it can play a part in flattening and directing the hair.

The second essential hairdressing tool is a pair of _scissors_, which in the present form emerged in the 14th century. The predecessors to scissors were shears, versions in gold having been found in Egyptian tombs. Again, this may have had some relation to the processing of wool. However, it seems likely that for everyday people, a sharp blade would allow hair to be hacked off.

Undoubtedly, the comb and scissors are the most important and basic tools of the hairdresser.

Washing hair would have been basic, and early soaps would have been made from wood-ash and animal fat. However, it seems more likely that people just did not bother to wash their hair, and would limit themselves to treating it with something like olive oil or butter. It is only in the latter part of the 20th century that chemistry has made reasonable shampoos available.

The purpose of *Styling* of hair is to make it more attractive or more practical. Men's hair was styled mainly to make it suitable for fighting or for labour. Greek soldiers cut their hair right back because, in battle, a forelock served as a useful handle for decapitating an enemy (hence the expression, to take time by the forelock).

For women, hair was the 'crowning glory' of Victorian times, which attracted the opposite sex or established her status with her own. Thus, although it was generally left to grow to its natural length, it was often gathered into some style using devices such as combs, pins, nets or head-ware or solutions of gums such as tragacanth which would keep it in place when dry. The attraction of female hair was believed to be such that maiden modesty sometimes required that it be covered, and in the case of nuns or girls with a strict religious upbringing (see the Girl with the Pearl Earring by Vermeer) it was tightly and completely enclosed. In other cases, it was permissible for unmarried girls to show their hair, but once married only the husband was allowed to see it. For this reason, some married women of the Orthodox Jewish faith wear a hair wig so that outsiders cannot see their real hair. In Jane Austen's time and later, married ladies wore a bonnet continually indoors as well as outdoors, to indicate their married status. The covering of hair by Muslim women is now well known.

The use of artificial hair in the form of wigs was an attempt to override the limitations of hair, as well as a hygienic device to avoid lice (the natural hair could be kept very short to facilitate de-lousing and the wig could be set aside at night). Another use of the wig was to create totally unrealistic hair styles, so big in some cases that the lady had to travel on the floor of her carriage. The hair of a wig could be treated in a way which was not acceptable to a human being. For example, the hair could be curled round a former, such as a rod or bone, and placed in an oven. The most that could be done with human hair was to place the hair in curlers, or in Victorian times, tying them with bits of rag and paper so that ringlets would be formed overnight.

Contemporary pictures suggest the following rough development of styles, in most cases, the hair retaining its natural length[3]:

1840 - 1852	Hair in dangling side ringlets, bun at back
1857 - 1865	Central parting, ears covered
1869 - 1881	Princess Alexandra style fringe, ornate, artificial hair,
1880 - 1890	Some fringes, often crimped
1900 - 1915	Hair high on head

Although the effect of heat on hair must have been known for a long time, it was in 1872 that M. Marcel in Paris invented the Marcel wave which used a pair of gas-heated tongs to crimp the hair. Skill was required to judge the temperature, one method being to test the tongs on a piece of newspaper (if it just charred, it was about right, which by later standards implies it was over-heated and probably damaged). He was also thought to be the first to have the idea of setting up a ladies' hairdressing salon. Before, no decent woman would have gone to a barber's shop, the only alternative being to have her hair done at home. Even so, the salon was not popular since "only women of a lower class" attended it, until it acquired some respectability and popularity later on. Thus Marcel can be thought of not only as the inventor of waving using heat but also as the originator of the ladies' hairdressing salon.

By the start of the twentieth century, the only alternative was to use relatively mild forms of curling by hand using suitable lotions (hand- or water- curling). This brings us closer to our story, which takes place between 1917 and 1939 - almost exactly the period between the two World Wars. The First or 1914 -18 World War not only sees the start of I. Calvete Ltd, but is pivotal to important social and technological changes.

Until then, women played a subsidiary part in society and were allowed in only certain activities. Strong social constraints ensured that the activities of married women were limited to the home and family. The war made such telling demands on man-power that women entered munitions and other factories in great numbers, where they earned more and worked better hours than when they were in service, one of the few employments previously available for uneducated single women. They were not about to give up this independence after the war and succeeded in getting the vote, albeit for women over 30. This new-found freedom extended to their hair, which may have been cut for safety reasons on the factory floor, and later developed into the post-war 'bob' - much to the disapproval of traditionalists. (This safety precaution was reflected in the second World War, when the US Government issued posters of the film actress Veronica Lake, whose trade-mark was long blonde hair hanging across her face, with the message that loose hair in the vicinity of rotating machinery was dangerous). It was only later that the ladies' hairdressing salon became popular, and after the war new ladies' hairdressing salons appeared everywhere, run by a new breed of hairdresser.

The war also gave some impetus to the technological or electrical fields. In 1860, Swan invented the incandescent electric lamp (20 years before Edison) and in 1897 he produced another model which improved on Edison's patented model. However, lamps were of little use without an external power supply and in 1883 Edison ran the world's first power station at Holborn in London, producing low-voltage, direct current. The first London power station comparable to a modern one was designed and built by de Ferranti at Deptford in 1891, which produced alternating electricity at 10,000 volts. The problems in establishing a convenient widely-distributed supply available to users such as hairdressers is well described in the reference[4] By 1900, there were 30 power stations in London which had risen to 70 at the outbreak of war. There was a confusion of supplies of both direct and alternating current in a range of voltages, and this was not rationalised until after the First World war.

In the early 20's, only 20% of households had an electricity supply and these were mainly in the urban areas. The main attraction of electricity was its superiority for lighting compared to gas, oil-lamps and candles, and this convenience was reflected in that electricity was supplied by a single cable to two meters, one for lighting and one for power. The light meter, taking advantage of the benefits of electric lighting, charged at a higher rate, and it was illegal to use the power line for lighting.

So during the First World War, the situation was roughly that industries might be using electricity as a source of power, and some privileged people were using it for lighting. Domestically, very little was used for appliances, and in trade, certain activities were contemplating the use of electricity, for appliances using motors or for heating. Electrical equipment was too expensive to be discarded readily, and with the shortage of spares caused by the war, there must have been a ready trade in electrical repairs and spares. It seems that hairdressers were certainly beginning to use electrical equipment, particularly hair-dryers, because my father was advertising a repair service for them in 1917.

The hairdressing business itself was on the verge of major developments. In about 1906, the first modern dyes were used for colouring hair, named Aureole by its originator, Eugene Schueller, and then later re-christened L'Oreal. And in 1906, as if standing in the wings, Karl Nessler in London demonstrated a machine which heated hair electrically in a controlled way, to create curls and the so-called the permanent waves. The first Nessler machine as it was called suffered all the faults of a prototype, - it was said to take 12 hours to do a 'perm' and consequently was very expensive - but it incorporated the basic elements that were to be developed later. Initially, the hair was also treated with caustic soda, which was bad for the hair and dangerous for the skin. In 1912 Nessler succeeded in overcoming the difficulty of tying a curler to the hair with his ratchet curler patents. By 1914 it had evolved so as to accommodate the long hair which was usual at the time by using long curlers. It is as well to remember here, that up to this time, apart from some possible 'tidying up', women's hair was left to grow long, even to its natural length, and so any styling was constrained to this condition. Thus, the Nessler system used very long curlers (originally, heavy metal rods) to cope with the long tresses being worn, which made the system very cumbersome.[5] It was a case of the technology adapting itself to the style. Later development of more efficient and shorter curlers would result in the hair styles we associate with the 20's and 30's.

Thus, by 1917, three strands of development had come together. Mains electricity was beginning to be available in homes and businesses. There was a demand for electrical products which could avail themselves of this. And women were beginning to have or expected shorter and wavier hair.

The origins of I. Calvete Ltd.

My father, Isidoro B. Calvete, founder of I. Calvete Ltd, was born in 1886 in a small village in Navarre, Northern Spain. At the age of 12, he was orphaned but he continued his education, and at an early age he became a travelling salesman for a large electrical wholesaler located in San Sebastian.

At this time, Great Britain was at the peak of its imperial glory while Spain had long descended from a similar peak. When our story starts, Spain had already been in decline since the Napoleonic occupation, and there were those who said that Africa started at the Pyrenees. The countries that once formed the Spanish Empire, particularly in the huge area from California and Florida in the North right through all South America, excepting Brazil, had successively declared their independence. The last of these was Cuba which revolted in 1895; when Spain tried to prevent this, the United States intervened in force by declaring war on Spain and in a sea battle in 1898 destroyed the whole Spanish fleet. Unable to supply its army in Cuba, Spain signed the Treaty of Paris and surrendered Cuba and gave sovereignty of Puerto Rico and the Philippine Islands to the United States. This was known as the year of the Great Disaster. There was a brief period of prosperity during the First World War when as a neutral, she became an important supplier of raw materials to the combatants, but then entered a decline in which half the population lived off the land. However, Spain managed to maintain some parity with the rest of Europe in technological developments, so that my father would boast that the small village where he had been born had electric street lighting before London. So by means of his evening school studies and representing a large wholesaler he was doing pretty well for his age and background.

However, his good luck did not last long. In 1908, because of an administrative anomaly, he was conscripted into the Spanish army; he must have made an impression with his then employers because they did everything they could to get him exempted so that they could retain his services, but without success. Perhaps because he was literate, compared to many of his colleagues, he became the commanding colonel's secretary. At the end of 1909, as a result of his privileged position, he discovered that an 'incident' was to be staged in Morocco and that his regiment was to be used in an unprovoked war of conquest in North Africa. As this conflicted with his principles, he decided to take the dangerous step of deserting and fled to France. As it happened, some 40% of his regiment was ambushed and killed in the outskirts of Melilla, on the Mediterranean coast of Morocco, which is still a Spanish enclave. This experience seems to have produced in him hereafter a strong antipathy to anything associated with war and anything military. Although he never declared it, I suppose he was a pacifist at heart.

Arriving at Paris, with my mother, he earned a living installing domestic and industrial electrical systems, at the same time advancing his studies. In the same year, my brother G. James Calvete was born. When the Great War started in 1914, my father's livelihood was assured, as most Frenchmen were being enlisted to face the German threat and to make up the huge losses on the Western front. Ironically, Spain never entered the War.

However, although the Calvete family was doing well in Paris, there was a constant threat from the Germans, and at one time they got close enough to Paris to shell the city. In spite of doing so well, my father decided, perhaps because my mother's brother was already living in London, to distance himself from the proximity of the war, and to leave France for England. In 1916, with whatever possessions they could take, my parents and brother James travelled to Dieppe to catch the cross-Channel ferry. However, they were detained at Dieppe for some time because the ferry they intended to catch, called the "Essex", had been attacked by a submarine.

1916. The incident of the "Essex" seemed a minor skirmish in the context of the war, but it had much wider implications. The "Essex" was an unarmed, passenger vessel which was torpedoed on the 24th March 1916 while on its way from Folkestone to Dieppe, by a German U-boat who believed it (allegedly) to be a mine-layer. It was carrying at least 325 passengers, some of which were American. About 80 persons were killed or injured, but the vessel did not sink and was towed back to Folkestone. (This was not the first such case – in May 1915, the "Lusitania", an unarmed liner, was sunk off Ireland with a loss of more than 1100 lives, 123 of which were Americans.) President Wilson protested vigorously and the Germans made the so-called "Essex Pledge" not to attack civilian vessels, but Germany renewed all-out submarine warfare to blockade Britain during which civilian vessels, some American, were sunk. These incidents played a large part in conditioning the American people to declaring war on Germany, which it did in April 1917 and was an important factor in Germany's defeat.

Wilson was associated with the "Essex" incident in another, more direct way. Two of the passengers on the "Essex" were Enrique Granados, *the Spanish composer and pianist, and his wife. Granados had premiered his new opera "Goyescas" in New York with such success that Wilson asked him to give him a piano recital in Washington. Consequently, he cancelled the berth he had reserved which was going directly to Spain and sailed later to Liverpool having to cross the Channel on the "Essex" to return to return home. When the ship was torpedoed, although he was safe on a life-boat, he saw his wife struggling in the water and jumped into the water to save her, but both were drowned.*

After waiting two weeks for the resumption of the service, the family finally sailed on the next vessel, the "Arundel" only to find that customs were turning back practically everybody because of the fear of spies. How my father, with no English and no Spanish documentation, only a French laissez-passer, managed to convince the authorities to let them through I do not know, but they did, and the family arrived in London on the 14th April 1916, with little money, no contacts and no English, and consequently my father had difficulty in finding work.. For a bit, he worked in a garage and then for a year at a company called "Synchronome" which manufactured accurate electrical clocks for world observatories and also master/slave clocks for large organisations such as railway stations, later supplying the then new Wembley Stadium. During this time, he helped found the Spanish Club at 5, Cavendish Square, W1, and which, incidentally, he completely re-wired. It became the focus of Spaniards and Hispanophiles living and working in London. The building was later occupied by the Spanish Chamber of Commerce, and now has been taken over by a smart private restaurant called "No. 5".

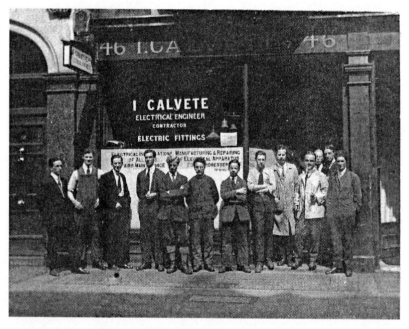

I. Calvete in 1917, at 46 Newman Street, W.1. My father is third from the left. The workers were probably men who had been exempted war service because of their nationality, physical condition or because they were conscientious objectors.

Finally, in June 1917, he decided to go into business for himself and he remained an entrepreneur for the rest of his life. He acquired premises at 46 Newman Street (which still stands today and is occupied by a beauty salon), near the junction with Goodge Street, a few minutes walk from Tottenham Road, and diagonally opposite the Middlesex Hospital. Newman Street runs parallel with Berners Street, in which were located the premises of R. Hovendens and Sons, major wholesalers for the hairdressing trade, so customers for one might pass the premises of the other. He went so far as to call himself a "Parisian Electrician". In addition, he put an advertisement in the Hairdressers' Journal since hairdressers had started using electrical equipment for massaging and hair-drying, and work started to flow in right away. The photograph suggests that he had made it into a Limited Company and had 12 employees. Because of the war-time shortage of manpower, he employed persons who were either unsuitable for military service or conscientious objectors who had refused to join up. In general, they knew little of electrical work and had to be trained.

The shop window displays "Electrical Installations of all kinds, Repairs, Maintenance", "Electrical Accessories sold here" and, most significantly, "Manufacturing and Repairing of Electrical Apparatus for Hairdressers". It was thus that hairdressing and hairdressing equipment was to become an important part of his business. Then, in 1917 two important events took place which were to play a large part in his future.

One day, a government official came into the shop with a problem. Because of the war, large amounts of correspondence had to be censored and certain documents had to be re-sealed with sealing-wax after inspection. Could a way be found to do this electrically, as the manual, time-honoured method with a taper was slow and rather dangerous? My father designed such a device and obtained a substantial contract. Perhaps this was his first attempt at inventing a new electrical device. More importantly, as a result of the contract, he was given a large number of blank, signed permits which enabled him to obtain strategic electrical materials which were difficult to get at the time and which were important for his repair work and for any development work he undertook.

The second event occurred later, but in the same year. The war continued with unabated fury in Flanders and elsewhere, but in London much business continued as usual. Towards the end of the year, a man came into the Newman Street shop with a problem. His name was **Eugene Suter**.

1918   Two historical events of great importance occurred in this year.   The United States, with a speed unexpected by the Germans, sent a million men to Europe to fight against Germany.   The German High Command, realising the parlous state of the civil population at home, and the hopelessness of the position now that the USA had entered the war, requested an Armistice for the 11th November 1918.   At the time, German troops, although in retreat, were still on French soil and no part of Germany had been occupied.   Consequently, the civilian population and the army were quite unprepared to accept that Germany had lost the war.   This was to lead later to a 'conspiracy theory' that the German Army had not lost the war but had been betrayed by certain factions (e.g. Communists, Jews,) and this would later lead to the rise of Nazism.   This was compounded by the Versailles treaty, signed in 1919, by which Germany had to pay huge compensations and concessions as Britain and France were determined that she should pay dearly for the consequences of the war.   The Germans particularly resented the "war-guilt clause" which was to fester for the next twenty years.

The second important event was the pandemic of so-called "Spanish Flu" which killed 200,000 people in Britain and was said to have killed world-wide more than those who died in the war, something between 25 and 50 million.   It was called Spanish only because the mortality was so great in Spain and this was well reported because being neutral, reports were not censored.   There is reason to believe that it started in the United States (where some 500,000 died) and was taken to Europe by the troops who travelled there in such large numbers, although it was first detected in a British Army hospital base in Northern France..   The cause was unknown at the time and caused panic because it could kill within 24 hours.   It was probably similar to avian flu which is why it causes such great concern today. Fortunately, none of my family were affected.

In Great Britain, women won the right to vote, but only if they were over thirty. Meanwhile in Russia, the Russian Revolution resulted in the Communist Party taking power; this would have important consequences for the next 50 years.

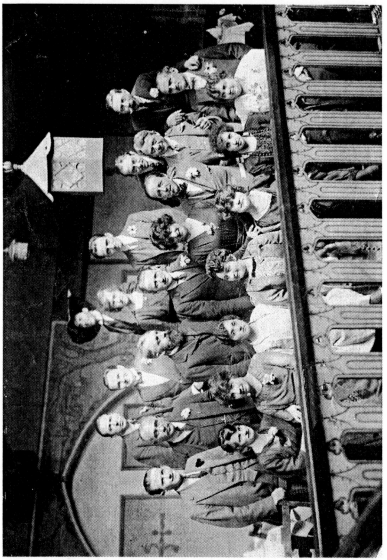

August 1919, a group of Spanish expatriates and wives in a London restaurant. My father is on the extreme left. The picture is of interest because the eight ladies all had "modern" hair styles which were greatly different to those before the First World War. Given the date, one supposes they were mainly Marcel waves.

The rise of Icall Ltd. (1917-1930)

Eugene François Suter was a Swiss national, who I shall call, as everyone else did, "Eugene", the founder of "Eugene Ltd". My father described him as the first inventor of a practical permanent-waving system, and as a consequence of their meeting, my father became the world's first full-scale manufacturer of permanent-waving equipment.

I have little to go on regarding Eugene's personality, but the impression I have is of a hairdresser in search of a product, with little technical knowledge but considerable commercial and hairdressing expertise, dare I say it, with a certain ruthlessness, - more of a "marketing" man than a "technical" man. How else would one explain that in a short time he managed to create an international reputation and business which placed the Eugene trade mark in the windows of so many hairdressers? To most women of the time, Eugene was synonymous with permanent-waving. His trade mark itself was brilliant, depicting an Arte Nouveau woman in the pose of an oriental goddess with eight heaters radiating star-like from the top of her head.

However, it was early days when he entered my father's shop in Newman Street in 1918. He was carrying either a Nessler heater or a drawing of one, and seeing the potential for such a device, he wished to have a design which was an improvement over the Nessler one, which was very heavy, slow and long, to cater with the long hair which still was common at the time. Also, about this time, Eugene had a theory that you needed two windings on each

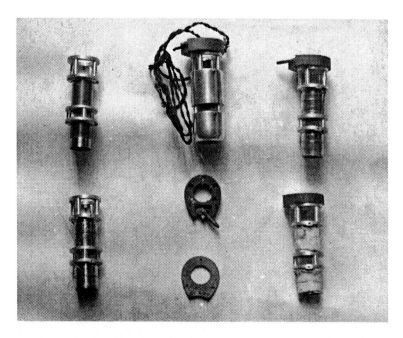

(Above:) An original photograph marked on the back "1918 Eugene Heater. Museum 4972." These are the prototypes of the Eugene Heater designed by my father and which were manufactured by him for Eugene for at least the next 10 years and are generally seen on photographs of so-called Eugene machines. The "Museum 4972" might puzzle some readers. At that time, telephone exchanges were operated by female operators and London was divided up into exchanges which received names which corresponded to the area, in this case, the British Museum (perhaps Eugene was staying in a hotel in that area). Another benefit may have been that an operator trying to memorise or write down a number before connecting to it, would find it easier to do so if it was a word and four digits, instead of seven digits. When dialling was introduced, the system was preserved, the digits on the dial also corresponding to letters of the alphabet, but the increase in demand in telephone numbers post-war resulted in a complete conversion to digits. These old numbers may be found in the pages of old telephone directories which are now available on the internet.

heater so that the hair near to the roots got hotter than the point end, because the thickness of wound hair was greater at the root end. He asked my father whether he could make one. At once, my father noted a number of serious faults with the design and created a heater of his own design. The heater was made from aluminium, for lightness, with sections cut from tubing. The spacers or 'legs" were fixed in holes in the rings. The upper part was of an unknown hard, thermal and insulating material (ebonite? – see opposite).

One of the problems at the time was that when a lock of hair was wound on to a curler, the part near the roots of the hair was thicker than at the other end. Apart from the hairs themselves being marginally thicker, each hair was of a different length, so the lock of hair tapered from the root end to the tip, and was correspondingly thicker when wound onto the curler. The taper could be natural, by the random breaking of hair on combing, or deliberate to achieve a smoother hair style. The thermal problem was resolved by using two electrical windings, the heater at the root end getting hotter than the other. This explained the unusual appearance of the heater which had a non-metallic ring at the upper end to allow the operator to handle the heater while it was hot, and an elaborate aluminium casting which held the two windings, connected by wires going through the spacers. Eugene took away the new design, tested it and ordered 1 gross at £1.03 each (modern value of about £40 each), which was possible because of my father's access to the necessary raw materials through the Government contract.

By 1918, orders of this size were being supplied to Eugene on a regular basis. Also, they had agreed on a design for curlers, which were supplied in batches of a 1000, in three lengths - 3½, 4 and 5 inches, and chandeliers with stands. An order for October 1918 showed that some basic problems such as the height of the stand were still to be solved and that demand was pressing:

"I am sending you a chandelier for you to see if same is alright. Will you please fix about five feet electric cord. The pole needs to two holes nearer the top, as the two already made makes the pole too short. Bearer will show where holes are to be made. Will you please let bearer know if we can have them back this afternoon, if so we will send for it, as it is wanted urgently to send to a customer. Please supply me with some adaptors with some solder on top, as they do not make proper connection. Eugene Suter"

Whether it was innocence on my father's part or astuteness on the part of Eugene, no mention was made of intellectual property. I doubt whether there was a contract signed, at least to start with, and my father was to regret that he neither patented the invention nor claimed licence fees, which would have been enormous in view of the numbers eventually sold. One machine could hold up to 24 heaters and the rest of the machine served to support the heaters over the head of the client and distribute electric power to them. It has to be realised that the design of the heater was essential for the success of the process. It is quite possible that neither of them had realised the implications of the invention and did not foresee that they would both be hampered by conflicting interests. Anyway, on 21st May 1918, Eugene Suter applied for US Patent 1,266,879 "electrical heating apparatus for permanently waving hair", although it could be said that he was only partly originator of the design, but it was obvious he already had his eye on world-wide applications. Later, Eugene was to make an appeal (which was upheld) against an infringement of this patent in the U.S.A., by the Nestle-Le Mur Company which had originated the idea of electrical waving before the war (Appendix 4).

(Opposite) A permanent-waving machine made by I. Calvete about 1920 for use and/or sale by Eugene. Note that the heaters are of the type shown in the previous picture which had been designed at Newman Street. It appears to have 22 heaters.

This classic design was to remain the basis of most permanent waving machines for the next 20 years, although improvements would be introduced in most aspects of it. It could be readily moved from client to client and the cords to the heaters not only provided the electric current but also took some of the weight of the heater.

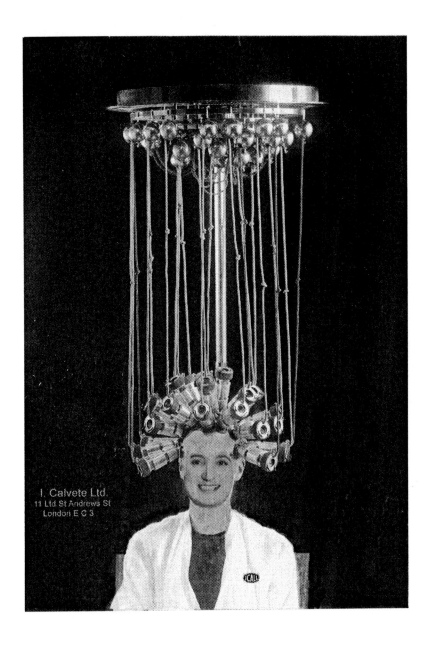

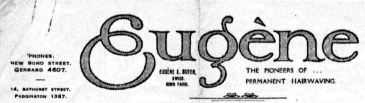

'PHONES:
NEW BOND STREET.
GERRARD 4607.

14, BATHURST STREET,
PADDINGTON 1387.

EUGÈNE E. SUTER,
SWISS.
BORN PARIS.

THE PIONEERS OF ...
PERMANENT HAIRWAVING.

NATURE'S BEAUTY REPRODUCED IN DETAIL.
Eugène's Implements are Fully Patented.

178, NEW BOND STREET, LONDON, W. 1, (Close to Old Bond Street).

14, BATHURST STREET, W. 2.

And 2, ST. ANN'S PLACE, MANCHESTER.

8th Oct. 1918.

ORDER GIVEN TO MR. CALVETE.

1 Gross of Complete Heaters as pattern, without casing *Covers*

@ 31/- each.

and not before.

DELIVERY:-   ⅓ Gross to be delivered within 1 month to 5 weeks, second ⅓ gross as required, but not to exceed 3 months.

MAISON EUGENE.

An order by Eugene for the earliest heaters, dated 8th October 1918. Under the heading Eugene, it says EUGÈNE E. SUTER, SWISS, BORN PARIS. Although being Swiss was quite respectable, it helped in hairdressing if you could claim some connection with Paris! The order is signed by the great man himself.

The order for one gross would mean the total order was worth £ 223.20, a sizeable amount in 1918 (equivalent to £9000 today?). An April order for 1000 curlers was at 3 shillings each, total value of £150.00

In a short while, the premises at Newman Street became too cramped for the production of heaters for Eugene and his own, plus the manufacture of medical and beauty equipment, so in 1918, the business was transferred to larger premises occupying the whole of the building at 11 Little St. Andrew Street, (which still exists in what is now known as Monmouth Street) a short distance East of Charing Cross Road and around the corner from the Ivy Restaurant. The display window shows little of interest except a hairdryer, but it retains the message "Electrical Machines for Hairdressers", and production soon required the leasing of rooms in adjacent buildings and even an assembly work-shop in Camden town and some premises in Clapham. The demand for heaters was now continuous, and together with the Everay High Frequency and other medical appliances and electrical repairs, the whole building was occupied with rooms in nearby buildings, some work being farmed out to Camden Town.

During this period, relations with Eugene were friendly, so much so that, while my family was living in Holland Park, Eugene himself came to the house to permanent wave my mother's hair in the kitchen one Sunday morning. Unfortunately, the stand for the machine was not available, so my father and brother had to hold up the chandelier for the hour that the process lasted. His diary for February 1921 showed that at that time he was costing the production of a new hair-dryer for Eugene.

This state of affairs soon changed. At the time, hairdressing machines were shown at fairs mainly run by engineering organisations such as the British Industries Federation. Hairdressing demonstrations and competitions were being run by a variety of unrelated organisations. My father entered a number of these and won first prizes in a series of them, both in Manchester and in London.

(Below) The larger premises (4 storeys) of I. Calvete Ltd. occupying the whole of 11 Little St. Andrew Street WC2, now Monmouth Street which runs into St. Martin's Lane in London near the junction with West Street, which enters Shaftesbury Avenue and Charing Cross Road, ca 1920. Even so, the whole building was insufficient and additional room was used across the road and at Camden Town. Today, the ground floor extending to the road junction to the left has been converted into a modern coffee shop.

The signs over the doors advertise Mazda electric light bulbs, which were still a bit of a luxury. Notwithstanding, the street light was an electric one, although parts of London were still lit by gas. It looks quite modern with clean lines, but retains the projecting rod just below the lantern which allows a ladder to be rested for maintenance.

John Logie Baird was at this time doing experimental demonstrations of his early television system and established a company called Television Ltd in an office in Upper St. Martins Lane - only yards away from the I.Calvete premises.

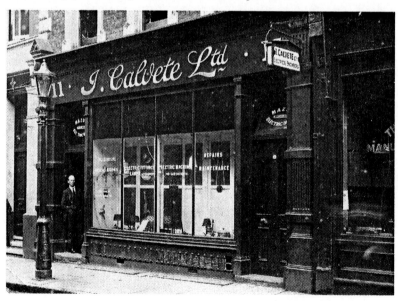

The crunch came at an exhibition, possibly organised by Dorland Advertising, at the Holland Park Skating Rink. Having again won several first prizes, the stand was crowded with hairdressers anxious to buy Icall equipment, but there was a stand-up row when Eugene came to the Icall stand and accused my father of competing with his own products and threatened him with breaking up the business arrangement if he persisted. An "agreement" was reached (24th March 1922) and thereafter, my father kept a low profile until the final break with Eugene took place in 1931. Until then he stuck to the manufacture of equipment for Eugene and dedicated his designing skills to electrical medical and beauty equipment.

These exhibitions were the forerunners of the annual Hairdressing Exhibitions held every year and run at that time by the Hairdressers' Wholesalers Association.

Meanwhile Eugene was having his own problems. Nessler had started selling its machines in Britain - whether these machines were manufactured in Britain or imported is not clear - and had accumulated a number of patents. Nessler had fallen foul of a Eugene heater patent in 1918, this time Eugene had infringed Nessler patent 23357 which was to do with curlers, specifically a curler with a ratchet which was quicker to use. A two page Nessler advertisement announced that a Justice Eve had found the case on their behalf and warned off any other copiers. To counter this, Eugene announced a modified version stating that "If holders of the original Eugene curlers would return them to I.B.Calvete, Little St. Andrew Street, the curlers would be altered by the omission of the ratchet and the substitution of the new mechanism, at the expense of Eugene Ltd." (HJ 26 Feb 1921 p. 405) This was a rare admission that his products were coming from elsewhere than his own factory, the existence of which seems to have been left to the imagination of the public. In fact, this new type of curler had been designed by my father and replaced the old system in which it was difficult to fix the hair to the curler, and was laboriously fixed with pieces of string. He was supplying them to Eugene at one (old) penny each! Of course, large numbers were needed and they were made in three lengths, the longest competing with the Nessler type which were still designed for the old-fashioned very long hair.

Following the row, it was decided that my father's direct sales activities would have to be restricted to markets abroad, so thereafter he maintained a low profile on the hairdressing side except at demonstrations where Eugene did not participate. This situation continued until 1930 when Eugene broke up the arrangement. Having established a manufacturing base, my father left the distribution to the company that Eugene had founded, apart from the occasional display of hairdressing items at exhibitions, but continued to supply Eugene in ever-increasing quantities. He designed a new improved heater in 1922 with an outer casing of aluminium and patented it in Germany and France, and was supplying Eugene with these at a rate of 500 per month and then 1000. Thus, one type of heater was being made for Eugene and another for his own machines. Another agreement was reached which arranged for a further 250 heaters per month to be supplied for the United States, at an agreed price of £0.75 (modern value of about £30). This confirms that Eugene was making inroads into the U.S. market, presumably competing against Nessler.

(Opposite) An advertisement (one of several pages) from the Hairdressers' Weekly Journal of 29th May 1920. From this we can now see that Eugene had patented the heater and was launching a permanent waving system – the Eugene system which was to become so famous. He gave the impression of making the equipment, which was in fact designed and manufactured by my father. Grafton Street is in Mayfair London., where Eugene had a hairdressing establishment which he presumably also used as a distribution system to market his system.

31

1922. Following continuous disturbances in Ireland, the Irish Free State was established, giving Southern Ireland a certain amount of conditional autonomy.. Mussolini marched on Rome, seizing power and establishing the first modern fascist state. This political model would be copied and developed later by Hitler. In Germany, the huge reparations demanded because of the War, had caused huge inflation so that money became worthless. The situation gets so bad that wages are paid as frequently as twice a day to give people a chance to spend them before the notes lose their value. Other countries agree to ease the burden of war reparations .particularly America who lends large sums to the Germans and unemployment and inflation began to fall. Conditions thus became less favourable for the Nazi party in Germany but it continued to be very active. Tutankhamen's tomb was discovered in Egypt.

Meanwhile, my father sought to diversify by seeking other small-scale applications of electricity which could be developed, and it was thus that he entered the medical and beauty fields, his main product being the Everay, a high-frequency device with glass electrodes, self-contained in a wooden carrying case which could be used for all kinds of ailments which would benefit by the stimulation of the local circulation of blood .

He also started selling hair-dryers to Selfridges, Gamages and other Department Stores and also opened an agency in Australia. Hair-dryers were the oldest of electrical hairdressing tools and were in demand for the home as well as for the salon.

My father was a great believer in publicity and he not only advertised regularly in the "Hairdressers' Journal" but became very involved in exhibitions. The first recorded case of exhibiting by I. Calvete Ltd was on stand 18 at an Olympia Health exhibition in 1923. In February of that year, Eugene returned from America and in the following month ordered 1000 heaters at £1.03 each. In 1924, an agreement was reached with Eugene, and relations were good enough for father to be invited to the Eugene Annual Dinner. Thereafter, there were frequent meetings with Eugene, and in April, my father went to Paris to visit clients. Eugene continued to visit the U.S.A., so his prospects there must have seemed promising. My father's diary says "The business was going well with good contracts from Eugene for permanent-waving equipment."

In 1923, business was doing well enough for my Father to buy a house in Wimbledon Park, SW18. In July, I was born in University College Hospital, Gower Street, London.

In May 1924, my father registered the trade marks ICALL (derived from **I. Cal**vete Ltd.), Teleswitch and Everay.

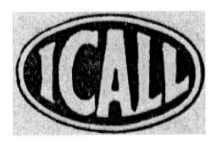

1925. Hindenburg was elected German president,

The most prestigious exhibition at which the company exhibited was the famous British Empire Exhibition of 1925, for which my father received a medallion. The stand in the photograph looks modest enough and concentrates mainly on the Everay equipment. However, it shows a rather primitive-looking permanent waving machine and also one salon hair-dryer and two hand hair-dryers. A couple of posters showing women's heads reveal the hairdressing connection.

In the same year, he also exhibited at the Daily Mail Ideal Home Exhibition, displaying two models of permanent-waving machine and hand-dryers. This time there were two machines, one of more advanced design and a wall model, and the same hand-dryers. In July, Eugene again sailed to the U.S.A. Meanwhile, my father obtained a French Patent 539749/20 for commercial use in France (Eugene was opposed to his selling in the United Kingdom).

Although the business was prospering, it was suffering from a lack of working capital. Materials had to be bought and employees paid, but relief appeared in the shape of an Argentine subject called Luis Navarro Viola who wanted to invest some venture capital. The sum of £6000 would today be equal to about £ 240,000 and so was a significant amount of working capital. On the 12th August 1926, an agreement was signed in which my father would remain Managing Director of the company. This injection of capital stimulated business and the collaboration with Eugene continued.

At home, my father was using his knowledge to improve our domestic technology. He constructed the first crystal set and then the first valve set in use in our neighbourhood. Our gramophone was, of course, an acoustic one, but when he finally bought one of the first commercial radios with a bakelite cabinet, he made a pickup for the gramophone so that it would play through the speaker. Of course, you still had to wind the turntable by hand.

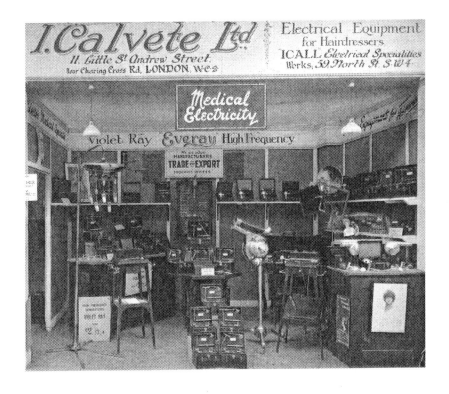

I. Calvete stand at the British Empire exhibition of 1925, dominated by the Everay High-Frequency machine. However, a simple permanent-waving machine can be seen on the left, with the heaters he had designed for Eugene and which were much smaller than the Nessler ones. In the middle, there is an early pedestal dryer, and on the right, some hand-dryers.

1926. In Britain, on the 4th to 12th May, after several years of industrial unrest, the General Strike took place. The miners, threatened by further wage cuts and longer hours, managed to get all major industries to come out on strike in sympathy, including all transport workers. With the Russian Revolution being so recent, there was a genuine fear of revolution. The Government recruited volunteers to supplement the services, and eventually the workers returned to work, excepting the miners who continued until August, but the slump was to continue until the 30's. My father during this period travelled to the factory by bicycle. First crude television transmissions by Baird.

By now, the premises at Little St. Andrew's Street were proving inadequate and some of the production and storage was transferred to new premises at Clapham, South London. (In 1930, all production would end up there.)

This year, my father became a British subject and took the opportunity of settling outstanding matters with the Spanish authorities regarding his desertion from the army 18 years before. In the same year, my brother James started work at Little St. Andrew Street at the age of 16.

In 1927, I. Calvete Ltd showed at an exhibition by the Federation of British Industry of which the company was a member. He also exhibited at the Daily Sketch Beauty Exhibition at Holland Park but, curiously, no hairdressing equipment was shown, except for hand-held dryers. However, a Eugene poster is clearly displayed on the wall, showing the classic Eugene mark.

Round about this time, my father must have become aware of the vulnerability of his position, because he had a single large customer, and if anything went wrong he would be reduced to his other sales which were through wholesalers direct to individual hairdressers. Although he advertised and exhibited at exhibitions, he would have to introduce a much more ambitious prizes, and reports and pictures of the winning styles invariably public relations exercise comparable to that used by Eugene.

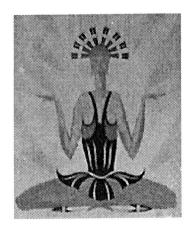 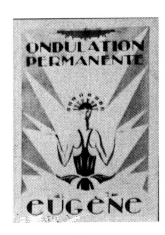

Two versions of the Eugene logo which were known worldwide.

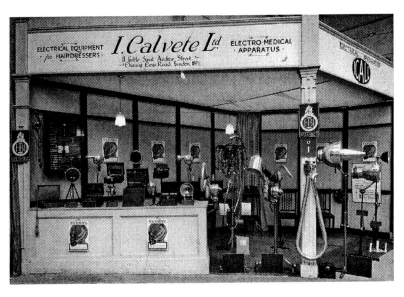

The British Industries Federation stand of 1928. To the left, the Everay equipment and to the right, the ultra-violet equipment. In the middle was the hairdressing equipment: a permanent-waving machine with 16 retractable tubular heaters which made the machine easier to use. Also some old-style dryers, though an early hood dryer can be seen.

This would have to include actual hairdressing demonstrations so that hairdressers could see what the equipment could do in practice, and to extend this to participation in hairdressing competitions. Competitions are more a test of the skills of the hairdressers involved, but there is no doubt of the prestige acquired by the equipment if it is consistently associated with the name of the maker of the equipment as well as that of the hairdresser.

1928. Voting by women extended to those over 21. Fleming discovers penicillin but fails to isolate it.

1929. After a decade of a bull market, the Wall Street stock market in New York crashed, initiating a period of depression until 1934, not only in the U.S. but in the rest of the world, with mass unemployment everywhere. In view of their own financial situation, the Americans called in their loans from Germany. The ensuing unemployment there, increasing from 1.25 million to nearly 4 million - 15% of the population, created a difficult situation there which greatly favoured the Nazi party.

About that time, I. Calvete Ltd opened a branch in Scotland and a factory in Germany (I. Calvete GmbH Frankfurt), and exhibited at the Leipzig Fair in 1927 and 1928. This seems to have been an attempt by my father to extend his influence beyond the Eugene sphere. By 1929, it was apparent that the German associates were swindling the company and an unannounced midnight raid was made to salvage all the important machine tools and cut losses and the German venture was abandoned in 1930. At the same time, attempts were made to extend the business to Belgium and Switzerland. Meanwhile I. Calvete signed a contract with Eugene for 5000 heaters a month at a price of 9/6 each (£ 0.48) which Eugene resold at 35/- (£ 1.75). It also included the provision of stands at £10. By now, machines were provided with 36 heaters, which enabled a whole head to be done in one go.

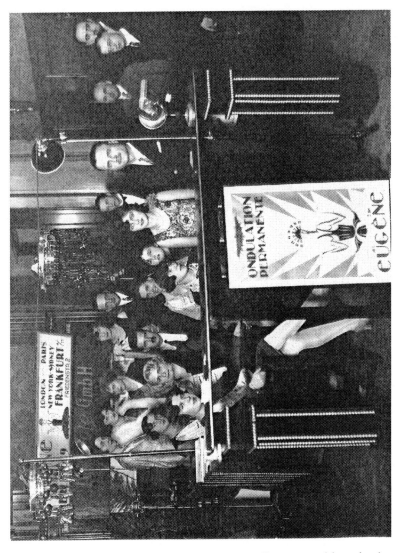

Frankfurt Exhibition stand in 1930. Two Icall p.w. machines in the back-ground and hand-dryer at the front. Note the hair styles of the German models and receptionist, presumably permanent-waved. The association with Eugene is shown by the sign at the back and at the front. The name I. Calvete GmbH is just visible at the back.

1930. Unemployment in Britain reached 2.6 million, causing great hardship because of the limited benefits available for the unemployed.

A new heater with improved insulation was patented and sent to Eugene. Although no problems had occurred with Icall heaters, there was always some concern by clients of the risk of an electric shock. It would be reasonable to say that standards of safety were not as high in those days, and in any case, the range of insulating plastics, that are taken for granted today, did not exist then. One solution adopted earlier by Icall was to earth the equipment, not necessarily a standard practice in those days, but this did nothing to allay the fears of the customer, so the alternative adopted (known as the 'wireless system') was to connect the heaters and then disconnecting them when applying to the curlers. A simple cord was used to take the weight of the heater, but the trouble was that the heater gradually cooled when applied, while the older heaters maintained a constant temperature, giving better control. But this was resolved by giving the heaters greater thermal capacity and the new machine was presented in November at that year's Hairdressers' Exhibition at Olympia. The method was known as the "falling heat" method because the temperature dropped when the current was disconnected.

The premises in Little St. Andrew Street had now become inadequate as record orders were being received from Eugene and as in March 1930, new premises were acquired at 59-61 North Street, Clapham, London SW4. These premises were an integrated factory and coped better with the increasing orders now made by Eugene not only for permanent waving machines but for other equipment such as dryers.

By now, "Eugene" was almost synonymous with permanent-waving and a name known nationwide to most urban women. As part of the social scene, in the hairdressing salons and on the streets, it looked as if was to be as permanent a feature as it was permanent in name.

*CHANGE OF ADDRESS

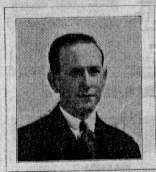

Mr. I. B. CALVETE, Managing Director.

ELECTRICAL SPECIALITIES

ICALL

Write now for Catalogue of "CHAMPION"&"CHAMPIONETTE" Pedestal Hairdryers, Central Hairdrying Installations, "Icall" and "Simplex" Portable Dryers, Pedestal and Portable Vibrators, "Everay" High Frequency, Curling Iron Stoves, Electrolysis, Radiant Heat Lamps, etc.

29th March, 1930.

We beg to advise our numerous customers and business friends that as from 31st inst. we are removing to

59/61, North Street, Clapham, S.W.4.

Owing to rapid extension it has been found necessary to centralise our business and equip Main Offices and Showrooms adjacent to our factory.

Our new premises are easily accessible. The nearest Tube Station is Clapham Common (6 minutes' walk, or 2 minutes by 177 or 77 'Bus). Telephone No.: Battersea 4634 (2 lines). Telegrams : ELECALVETE, CLAPCOM, LONDON.

The House of Calvete has long been recognised in the foremost rank for service and dependability of apparatus for the Hairdressing profession.

" ICALL " Products are the outcome of specialisation ; they " build business " and give complete satisfaction to your customers. The whole range of Hairdressers' Electrical Equipment is manufactured at our own factory, which is the largest of its kind in Europe. Your further co-operation, enquiries, and orders will be esteemed. Our expert representatives are always at your service.

" ICALL " Electrical Equipment has been adopted by the best establishments all over the world.

" I C A L L " P R O D U C T S MEAN
SERVICE AND DEPENDABILITY.

DAILY MAIL
IDEAL HOME
EXHIBITION
OLYMPIA

Stand No. 432
Gallery, Main Hall

I. Calvete Ltd.,
59, North Street, London, S.W.4.

'Phone :
BATTERSEA
4634—2 lines.
Telegrams :
ELECALVETE,
CLAPCOM,
LONDON.

The move to Clapham. Note that although Permanent-Waving Equipment was the most important item being manufactured, it is barely mentioned in the advertisement.

The intermediate years (1931 - 1935)

In 1931, as a member of a team headed by Lord Rootes, my father travelled to the British Empire Exhibition in Buenos Aires in Argentina, where he exhibited his products and established an agency. Because sea-travel was the only practical form of transport, this meant an absence of more than three months. He had cavalierly announced his business journey in the Hairdressers' Weekly Journal (...and now to South America), and stated that Icall was the only British firm in this line to exhibit, "but we have every confidence that our products will uphold British prestige for sound design, expert workmanship and attractive and beautiful finish". However, Eugene took the opportunity of his absence to sever the relationship which had lasted so long. On his return, he went to Eugene's for "final ending of the working arrangement as their manufacturers" in June. Presumably Eugene had acquired a factory (in Hendon, London) started to manufacture their own equipment and had acquired the technology necessary to be independent. This meant that I. Calvete Ltd was left only with its direct sales, which had been inhibited while Eugene called the tune. A new phase was beginning. At least now he was free to compete openly in his own right.

Although the Clapham factory was now working full tilt and had its own showrooms, in 1932 a showroom which overlooked Shaftesbury Avenue, was opened in Central London at 52 Dean Street which was retained for 5 years.   Momentum was also maintained by presenting permanent waving demonstrations around the country to show hairdressers how to use Icall equipment.

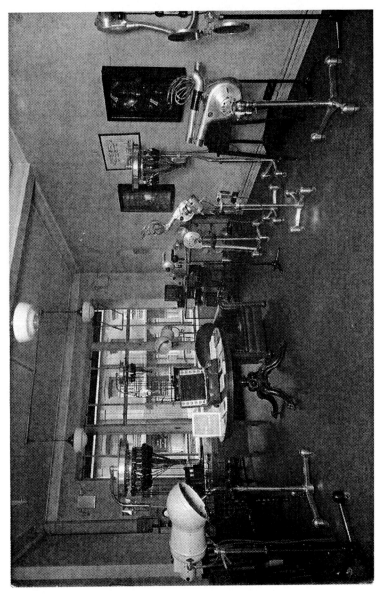

The showroom at 52 Dean Street. The window at the end overlooks Shaftesbury Avenue. As well as showing the range of Icall products, numerous demonstrations were held here as well in other parts of the country.

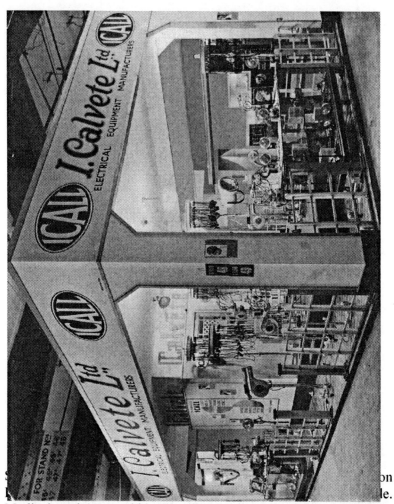

on
le.

Medical equipment, although still manufactured, hardly featured in this stand. No less than six permanent waving machines were shown, together with a range of dryers, from the old models to tubular canopy types and the first modern suction dryer. A new hand-held dryer which blew air over a wider area rather than a strong jet, also put in an appearance. This was the first exhibition in which my father was freely able to promote his own equipment.

1932, unemployment in the U.K. reached a peak of 2.8 million.

My father designed a new croquignole heater which he patented. Business, which had dropped off after the Wall Street crash, was now doing extremely well and beating all records (in November alone, there were more than £3,200 of orders, or approximately £ 120,000 in today's money) and many came in as a result of the Fair of Fashion Hairdressing Exhibition in September. The factory was extended to include the ground floor. A stand was taken at the Brussels Fair.

In 1933, Hitler, who now had the support of German industrialists (who feared the communists) and of perhaps 30% of the population, was reluctantly appointed Chancellor by Hindenburg on the 30th January, under the illusion that he could be controlled by other members of the cabinet. This was the point of no return which would lead to the Second World War.

At the 1933 British Industries Fair at Olympia the new Excelsior (later changed to Velox) dryer was shown for the first time. Company staff had reached the 100 mark. Demonstrations at Dean Street were very successful. The Excelsior dryer was improved by using ball-bearings. About this time, J. Bari-Woolls joined the company as a consultant and drew large crowds of hairdressers to Icall hairdressing demonstrations

Eugene continued to demonstrate his skill at public relations by means of an extensive and continuous publicity campaign in newspapers and journals, and even making short films that were shown in towns all over the country. In October, he took a full page advertisement in the Daily Mail, claiming to be the "Perfecters of the Permanent-Wave". Eugene thus became by far the best known source of permanent waving and was reputed to have 15,000 registered hairdressers users of Eugene equipment. Papier mâché models of the Eugene trade mark inscribed "Registered Eugene Waver" were distributed for display in salons, but the prestige of using the name in hairdressers' businesses entailed a number of obligations enforced by Eugene. In general, this meant that if the name Eugene appeared anywhere in the hairdresser's premises or advertising, it meant that Eugene equipment and materials had to be used. Unidentified inspectors would travel round the country checking that this was so, and prosecutions could ensue. A particular check was kept on the use of sachets (q.v.)

1934. In Germany, on the 2nd of August 1934, Hindenberg died and Hitler makes himself Dictator (Fuhrer) with a single-party (Nazi) system. The Reichstag was closed and elections were abolished. The beginning of persecution of the Jewish population and rearmament.

This year I. Calvete Ltd exhibited at the B.I.F. Fair in Birmingham and at Olympia in London (Sep). The stand was deemed the most original of the show and won second prize. Business was recovering from the depression and during the last quarter, the company had a turnover of £18,000 (equivalent to about £ 720,000 today). The business appeared to be flourishing on all fronts, perhaps the best results the business had ever had. Considerable effort went into giving demonstrations at which Bari-Woollss was much sought after for technical advice.

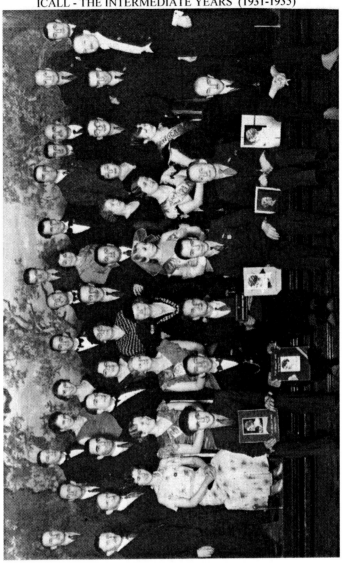

An Icall demonstration in East Ham on January, 1934. At the back, with bow-ties, my brother and father. Lower down, the Lady Mayoress with models each side with hair which has just been styled, wearing Icall sashes. The gentlemen in the front row were the hairdressers, except the one holding a box marked "Hairdressers' Orphans Fund".

The Picture House, Bridge Street
WALSALL

Tuesday 13th March at 7.45 p.m.
The Victoria Hotel
WOLVERHAMPTON

Wed. 14th March at 3 & 7.45 p.m.
Imperial Hotel, Temple Street
BIRMINGHAM

Thursday 15th March at 7.45 p.m.
King's Head Hotel
COVENTRY

All above Demonstrations will be followed with
a lecture by J. Bari-Woollss

DAILY DEMONSTRATIONS
Morning and Afternoon at our Showrooms

The Icall is the most advanced system which can be relied upon to produce perfect results in a minimum of time; it is very economical in its initial and running costs.

I. Calvete Ltd.

Specialists in the manufacture of Permanent Waving Equipment of the highest class and quality for nearly 20 years.

Headquarters:
ICALL WORKS,
North St., Clapham,
London, S.W.4.

Showrooms:
52, Dean Street,
Shaftesbury Avenue,
London, W.1.

Typical advertisement in a 1934 Hairdressers' Weekly Journal for Icall demonstrations. Evening classes were also given at Birmingham, Manchester, Preston, Liverpool, Nottingham, Sheffield, Leicester, Glasgow, Cardiff, Leeds, Newcastle, Bristol, Plymouth, Dublin, Belfast and Southampton. (Courtesy of Hairdressers' Journal International)

48

1935 Italy invades Abyssinia (today Ethiopia).

Eugene introduced a policy of price fixing which temporarily affected Icall sales. However, Icall developments continued with the launch of a new sachet, and in April the launch of a new line of hair dyes called Velox Patent, and a new curler called Presto.

By now, Eugene claimed to have its own factory making equipment and changed the name of the company from Eugene Ltd. to Suter Electrical Ltd. Drawings of an immense factory appeared in the Hairdressers' Weekly Journal but, by and large, Eugene advertisements nearly always gave just the West End address - 15/16 Burlington St, London W.1. I recall mention being made of a factory in Hendon and some advertisements did include a factory address: Eugene Works, Edgware Road, Hendon, N.W.9. This part of Edgware Road is some 10 miles from where this road joins Marble Arch. However, Kelly's Post Office Directories for the 30's do not show any premises in Eugene's name.

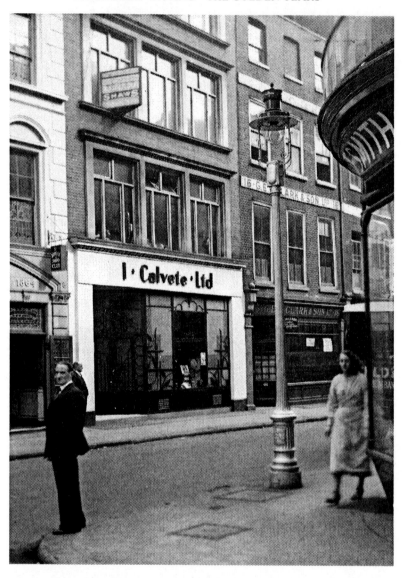

The showroom (Icall House) in 15 Greek Street, London which lies west, and runs parallel, to Charing Cross Road, and was used from 1937. The first floor was fitted as a salon which was used for hairdressing demonstrations. The design of the Art Deco frontage was also used in Icall catalogues and letter-headings.

Icall - The final years (1936-1939)

1936. In February, elections in Spain were won by the Popular Front and the formation of a new republican government. July outbreak of Spanish Civil War, caused by insurgency of right-wing military groups against the democratically-elected, left-wing Republic. Daily news of the war became a constant concern at home. Franco was declared chief of state. Germany and Italy formed the Berlin-Rome Axis or fascist alliance. Accession and abdication of Edward VIII and marriage to Mrs Wallis Simpson, an American divorcee. They assumed the title of Duke and Duchess of Windsor.

This was a year of crisis, both nationally and for the company. Mr Viola who had financed the company since 1924, had decided to retire and wanted his original investment back. Although business was good, finances became critical and some company shares had to be sold. The situation was aggravated when, after sacking the work's manager because of his unpopularity with the staff, he started rumours in the trade that Icall was going bankrupt. As a result, it was difficult to get credit, and creditors became concerned and applied pressure by insisting on payment on delivery of materials. An entry in my father's diary says "We fear that unless Eugene comes to our rescue, we might not survive." There was a strong probability that the company would go under even although the business was thriving. In fact, business was going incredibly well, sales surpassing £5000 (equivalent to £200,000 today) per month, and demand for sachets was greater than production, all of which required new premises in Lillieshall Road round the corner from the factory. It is not clear from whence the initiative first came, but Mr. John Bunford, Managing Director of Eugene, arranged for a meeting on the 24th March at the Mayfair Hotel for negotiations with Eugene Suter. An agreement was signed in April that Eugene would take control of I. Calvete Ltd, and that my father and Viola would lose their preference shares and life directorships but that creditors would be paid in full. My father continued as managing-director but lost overall control. Manufacture of some of the products was taken over by Eugene. There was a demonstration of a new wireless permanent waving machine Sales increased and the factory could not keep up with orders for sachets and Perfex dryers.

During 1936, Eugene and Co. became a public company and the running of the company was taken over by a Board of Directors, although some old hands, such as Bamford, remained many of the Board seemed to have little knowledge of the hairdressing business. Eugene himself seemed to take a back seat, quite possibly because he was suffering from ill-health. Relying heavily on its large base of established professional customers in many of the salons of the country it indulged in extravagant publicity addressed at the general public, such as sending models with Eugene perms and in bathing costumes to sea-side resorts where they would parade on the beach or in the water. They also had a synchronised swimming team which displayed at public swimming pools, film clips of which are available on the internet.

(Opposite) To counter the publicity of Eugene which had become so intense, in October 1936, I. Calvete Ltd presented its most ambitious stand ever at the Hairdressing Exhibition at Olympia, which won first prize for its originality and had cost £1300 (£ 52,000 pounds in today's money). According to my father's diary, the sales it produced justified the expense. The end of the long stand had a rotating turntable so that three models could be displayed alternately. See also photograph on next page.

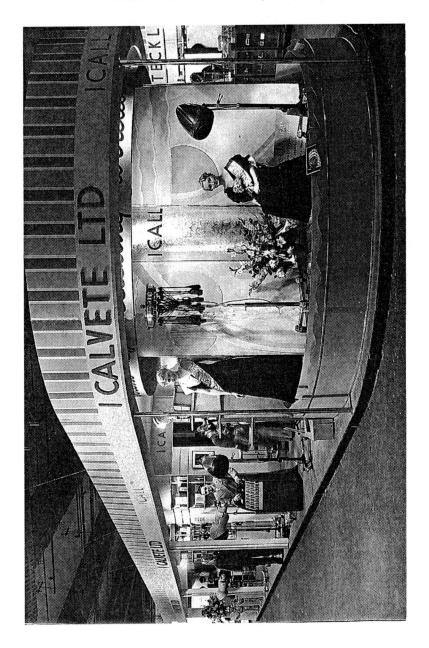

The civil war in Spain and its associated European politics were to have an increasing effect on my father. The origins of the war were complex but, to simplify, Spain was in the power of the army and of the church and the ever-greater backwardness of the country meant that when a left-wing government acquired power, some of its supporters indulged in excesses. This gave Franco an excuse to start an uprising on the 18th July, on which day a cousin of mine was killed in the street in San Sebastian. As has been stated earlier, my father in his youth deserted the army, so it was not difficult to see which way my father's sympathies lay.

On the last day of the year, Bari-Woolls resigned. Since he had joined the company he had not only done a great deal to increase knowledge on the principles of permanent-waving but he had imparted this knowledge to many hairdressers all over the country and even abroad at the demonstrations regularly run by the company to instruct hairdressers. He was a regular contributor to the "Hairdressers' Journal" and was thus widely known, so that his presence at the Icall stand at exhibitions, giving demonstrations and consultations, always resulted in a large crowd at the stand. A number of personal reasons for his resignation were responsible, but he was doubtless tempted by the opportunity to assume the editorship of the second edition of "The Art and Craft of Hairdressing" on the death of the previous editor and author, G. A. Foan, the previous year. This 620-page volume is a treasure chest of information on pre-war hairdressing which is perhaps not better known because its publication date was close to the start of the war.

1937. The civil war in Spain was gradually turning in favour of Franco, assisted by the Italian Army and the German Air force who used the war as a practice ground for the coming conflict. This included the notorious bombing of the Basque capital Guernika on market day, a purely civilian town with no military importance, which was to become the forerunner of Warsaw, Amsterdam, Coventry and London. The Italians also sent 50,000 "volunteers" from their army. Meanwhile, Franco had the advantage of having most of the army on his side and much of the arms. The Republic had to resort to arming the workers to form militias.

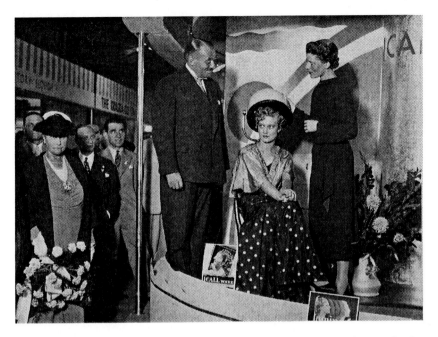

Hair and Beauty Fair, Olympia, October 1936 - the rotating end of the stand.

The picture shows a close-up of the turntable, with a model, wearing a short protective cape, sitting under a suction dryer. The two persons inspecting her are of interest.

The man was Mr Ernest Brown, Minister of Labour of the Baldwin and later Chamberlain Cabinet. He later became Minister of Agriculture and Minister for Scotland. The young lady on the right of the model was Miss Golden Voice, or Jane Ethel Cane, who by winning a speech contest, recorded the voice for the first talking clock which was in use by the Post Office from 1936 to 1963 and thus became a well known personality. By dialling TIM, you could hear her voice telling you the exact time. Her voice can still be heard on a site on the internet.
(web.ukonline.co.uk/freshwater/clocks/ spkgclock.htm)

Meanwhile, Britain and France adopted a non-intervention policy, so the only outside help came from the purely volunteer International Brigade, made up mainly of working-class people and idealists from many countries; the Soviet Union also assisted but only to fulfil their own ends. All the gold reserves were taken from Madrid to Moscow Coronation of George VI. Basque children arrive from Bilbao to escape bombing. Mitchell, designer of the Spitfire, dies.

A lease was signed to use 15 Greek Street in Soho, as a Show Room, which was also used for hairdressing demonstrations. Business continued hesitant because of the international situation, and my father was by now thinking of alternatives to the hairdressing business. He even considered the possibility of selling up and starting a hotel in London for continental people.

Although my father had sent some help to members of the family in Spain, a more direct emotional contact now arose. Franco had now surrounded Bilbao, important for its steel and arms manufacture. The position of the civil population, both from the food and safety points of view, was now dire and a decision was made to evacuate the children, (an action similar to that during the war when evacuee children were taken out of London). Of some 10,000, 3840 Basque children, 95 teachers and 120 female workers were assigned to England and they sailed on the 23rd May, crowded together, in a ship called the "Habana". The British Government did not oppose this, but provided no help apart from protecting the vessel from attack, so provision was made by a committee of volunteers. After landing at Southampton, they were taken to North Stoneham nearby, where tents had been set up in afield. I was later told by one of the children that after starving in Bilbao and having nothing to eat on the ship, they were greeted at the camp with thin cucumber sandwiches, something they had never seen before.

My father's diary says he left home at 7:20 and arrived at the camp at 9:40. "Worked very hard and got wet to the bones. Car break down and spent the night at Winchester." From Stoneham, the children were distributed to some 94 large houses which held some

30-100 children each, situated all over the country. My parents established a strong relationship with groups situated at Barnet, Theydon Bois, Carshalton, Kingston and Putney. On the 20th June, Bilbao fell, news which brought intense despair to all the children, whose future was now in question, as there was little likelihood of an early return.

Sales were down due to the dislocation of sending some of the production to the Eugene factory at Hendon and the move to new showroom at Greek Street.

1938. In March, Hitler occupied the whole of Austria and made it part of Greater Germany. In October, he occupied part of Czechoslovakia after signing the infamous Munich Treaty with Britain and France, in which Czechoslovakia was disposed of without consultation. Later, he occupied the rest of that country in spite of saying that he had no more territorial ambitions. Towards the end of the year, the Spanish Civil War gradually coming to an end with the capture of Barcelona.

In 1938, the Hairdressing Exhibition at Olympia although well attended was a commercial failure due to international tension, though Icall won prize for best stand. Rumours have spread that Eugene have stopped making Icall products because of the recession.

Notwithstanding, Eugene with its new administration threw itself wholeheartedly into publicity - whether this was due to great optimism or because sales had gone down drastically, it is hard to tell. In January particularly big advertisements were placed in the daily newspapers. They had also made a number of films comparing old-fashioned styles with the new Eugene "authentic" permanent-waving. In the HJ, double-page adverts announced that Eugene had 15,000 hairdresser clients, that they were going to increase production and their sales-force to meet the demand. The adverts pointed out that only Registered Eugene wavers could benefit from the new Engineering Service. Great stress was placed on the fact that the name Eugene could only be used when using

Eugene equipment and sachets. Even, a two-page advertisement written in 1920 by Eugene giving his theories on waving was re-published several times.

The wave of enthusiasm indulged in by Eugene overflowed into an advertisement in the Hairdressers' Journal of January 1938 which showed an artist's impression of the Eugene factory at Hendon. One is tempted to believe that it includes some artistic licence as well.

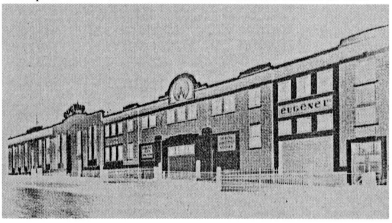

Beneath, it says:

"Time has proved the Eugène Method and the Eugène principles of Permanent waving indisputably correct.
Today the ideal Method is one that produces Permanent waves and curls that satisfy your customers and at the same time provides for you a continuous all-the-year-round business
In brief, the ideal Method is the Eugène method...the Method your customers know and prefer...the Method that is nationally advertised and for which there is a continuous, steady, all-the-year-round demand , the Method that has behind it the largest and most efficient organization of its kind in the world."

In November, at the Annual General Meeting at which Eugene Suter was present, I. Calvete was re-elected Director. However, my father was now convinced that there was no stopping Hitler and that war was inevitable. He made secret plans for us to emigrate to Ecuador in South America with another Spaniard and his family.

The family by now had formed strong friendships with the Basque children and their teachers and many of the latter were invited to Greek Street to have their hair permed. Also my father organised a number of concerts at halls in various parts of London in which the children in Basque costumes sang and danced, to raise money to supplement that voluntarily given by the public. Moves were started in Spain to have them repatriated and eventually some 3000 went back in batches. However some of them decided to remain in this country and stayed on during the war, eventually becoming British citizens. Some of the houses at which they had originally stayed were later to have blue plaque attached to them to commemorate the fact. (Ref. 23)

1939   Britain and France recognise Franco's government. Czechoslovakia ceases to exist as such.   On the 31st March, the civil war in Spain ends, and Franco remains dictator for another 36 years. Florey and Chain isolate penicillin and thus initiate antibiotic therapy.

My father now, concerned and disillusioned by the international situation, started to look for alternatives.   For commercial and family reasons, he decided to resign from I. Calvete Ltd and emigrate.   Thus on the 31st March (ironically, on the day the Spanish civil war ended) he formally resigned from I. Calvete, which would become absorbed by Eugene; he also requested measures to be taken to protect the employment of staff. The staff were of course shocked by this development and thought he was going to set up another business elsewhere, prompting some to ask to be employed by him.   My education was abruptly stopped at school.   Having sold his house, car and furniture, on the 17th June, my father and mother and I set sail from Liverpool to South America.

September. Germany invades Poland   Britain and France declare war on Germany thereby starting the Second World War.

Schematic representation of cross-section of hair.

↑ To ends of hair ↑

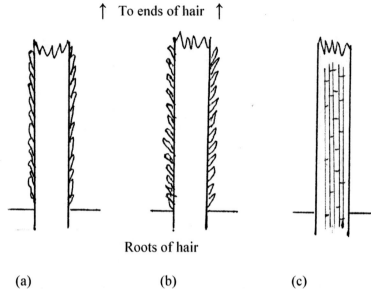

Roots of hair

(a)   (b)   (c)

(a) Dry, neutral hair with scales lying close to the body of the hair. Such hair is easier to comb from root to tip, and this is also helped by the cuticle scales protruding as little as possible and lying towards the point.

(b) Shampooed hair. Alkalinity will tend to make the scales open and protrude, water will have a similar but smaller effect. The hair surface is rougher, more difficult to comb and more likely to tangle.

(c) The central part of the hair consists of long chains of keratin which are aligned with the direction of the hair. These chains are linked one to another by chemical links at various points along the chain. This makes the hair more rigid and retain its shape, whether straight, waved or curly, so that attempts at simple physical change are only temporary. If the links can be broken and, preferably, rejoined in the new configuration, the new shape can be considered "permanent". Incidentally, scales act as a water-proof shield for the hair, so opening them is desirable to facilitate access by chemicals to the central keratin chains.

The Nature of Hair and Water

Human hair is not fundamentally different to the hair or fur of other mammals. It has presumably evolved so that the body can retain heat, although on the head it may also have played a part in reflecting intense sunlight such as that to which early man may have been exposed in South Africa, particularly after adopting a walking posture. I am not sure it is clear why parts of the human body have lost their hair, but because of clothing we can for practical purposes say that hair is generally only visible on the head and, in males, on the face.

The composition of hair is also not very different to that of skin or nails, being made of a protein called keratin, but it is formed in a very different way, being extruded from follicles in the skin as a long, thin cylinder. In structure it is a bit like a tree, where its constituent molecules of keratin form chains which are aligned in the direction of growth while the outside of the hair is covered in scales which also follow the direction of growth. In addition, these chains have links between them, rather like struts, which make the hair resist permanent deformation.

If the hair emerges from the follicle uniformly it creates a straight hair. However, if for genetic reasons a degree of eccentricity is present, that is, the hair grows faster in one part of the follicle, the hair will emerge curled, giving either slightly wavy hair or tight curls. The latter, with black hair, probably gives some protection from intense sunlight. Where the climate is more moderate this is less of a requirement, the hair may be straight and/or fair.

The colour of hair is also determined by genetic factors and can only be changed externally by bleaching or dyeing. The amount of pigment in hair decreases with age and ends up being grey or even white.

Recent academic work carried out by L'Oreal in 2003 and which has practical significance for the practising hairdresser is Reference 17, which is a comparative study of Asian, Caucasian and African hair - of particular interest in a multi-cultural society. It was found that there was little chemical difference between the three types but considerable physical differences. African hair has the appearance of a twisted oval rod, while the others were nearer to circular. Asian hair has a greater diameter. There were differences in water absorption as well. When immersed in water, the radial swelling of all three reaching a maximum after about 100 minutes. However, Caucasian hair levelled off at about 10%, Asian at about 8.5% while African saturated at about 7%. [Theoretically, if certain assumptions are made, the final water content of the hair would be 25%, 22% and 19% respectively). This shows that for some reason African hair is dryer than the others and also that hair can contain quite a lot of water after shampooing even after the surface moisture has been removed. For whatever purpose, this can slow down the absorption of chemicals as solutions.

The relative strength of the three types of hair was also examined. African hair was found to be more brittle than the other types, and together with its greater curliness, combing results in breaking the hair into pieces rather than taking out a few, whole strands.

The styling of hair generally requires the waving or straightening of hair. The latter involves the same principles as waving although the result is the opposite of waving. Waving implies some deformation of the hair, but as hair is an elastic material it has a tendency to return to its natural form unless something is done to make the deformation permanent. The processes that can be used to make the hair more amenable to permanent deformation can be classed as: none, moisture, heat, chemical products and a combination of these.

The first of these is represented by the papers Victorian ladies tied into their hair on retiring or more recently by curlers which are left in for a long time in the hair. No heat or moisture is used and obviously this was anything but permanent since the natural elasticity of the hair would return it to its original condition.

Water alone was used in what was called water-waving. This too has a low level of permanency although it can be made longer-lasting by the use of additives to the water which keeps the setting in position. This is not to be confused with what is now called setting which is carried out on hair which has already received some curling treatment. In the early days, the setting solution was generally a viscous solution which held the hair in place generally containing gum tragacanth as an adhesive and glycerine to prevent total drying, but today there is a wide range of products as creams, lotions and aerosols. However, one shampoo will generally destroy the setting of the hair.

To understand the principles of permanent waving, a little elementary chemistry/physics is necessary. The molecules of keratin which make up the hair are like chains which are aligned with the shaft of the hair. These chains are linked together by quite short little links, in fact they are two sulphur atoms that look a bit like : — S — S — . These strengthen the hair and make it tougher. The trouble is that at the same time, they prevent the hair from changing its shape, a) if you are trying to straighten it, or b) when you are trying to wave it. So the way forward is to break the link between the two sulphur atoms which allows you to accomplish either the straightening or waving. Once this is done, ideally you should join up the sulphur links again in their new configuration, to achieve a permanent effect. To break the links in the first place, there are three main methods. First, the brute force method of heat alone. Second, assisting heat with water or better still, adding a chemical additive such as borax or ammonia, to the water, which is the method used in classic permanent waving. The third is using a purely chemical method (cold-waving) which adds a hydrogen atom to each sulphur atom and breaks the link, and removing the hydrogen atoms when you have finished to make the effect permanent.

The use of heat alone goes back to the days of Marcel waving, although the technique survives even today in the heated styling brushes which are readily available for home use. The process is one in which the hair is softened rather like a piece of plastic which then sets in its new position.

Another analogy is the ironing of a wrinkled garment with a hot iron. There is probably some residual stress in the hair which tends to return it to its original form because the cross-links between the chains of keratin are still in their original position.

This thermal process can be enhanced by the presence of water, which is converted into steam. Hence, some of the old permanent-waving literature refers to "steaming-time". Steam not only increases the plasticity of the hair, but also improves the transfer of heat and avoids general or local over-heating which can damage the hair. While there is water present, the temperature can hardly go over 100°C, and thus affords some control over the temperature. To extend our previous analogy, it is rather like ironing a wrinkled garment with a steam iron.

Even the steaming process will hardly affect the cross-links between the chains of keratin and this can only be done by the addition of certain chemical products to the water, which made waving truly permanent. In general, these were fairly simple materials, but their nature was a closely guarded secret and their sale a profitable source of income. From the start, therefore, chemicals would be applied to the hair to achieve this effect; they would generally be in the form of solutions in water, which in the trade acquired the name of "reagents". Much of this work was empirical, that is, people tried out various chemicals and some of these proved at least partially effective. Examples of such chemicals are ammonia (in the form of ammonium carbonate), sodium sulphite and borax which are alkaline. Ammonia had the advantage of being a gas, so it was easily removed on concluding the process. Although these products were often sold as solutions, it became convenient to supply the chemical in special porous sachets which were moistened and then wrapped around the lock of hair before applying the heater and steaming.

Then, we come to the use of chemical products which require little or no heat. These simply open the cross-links between the chains of keratin which makes the hair soft and easily curled and the cross-links are reconnected in their new positions by the use of another chemical product (a neutraliser, such as hydrogen peroxide) to produce a cold permanent-wave.

It is useful to consider the part played by water in all parts of the hairdressing process. Hair can absorb a certain amount of water, more so if alkaline, which makes it swell slightly and makes it more plastic and the surface scales open so that the surface becomes rougher. The process is reversed on drying and the scales will close, more with an acidic solution, making the hair smoother.

The relevance of the pH (or acidity/alkalinity) of water on hair can be summarised by the following scale:

pH	**less than 7**	**<**	**7**	**>**	**more than 7**
	Acid		**Neutral**		**Alkaline**
Everyday examples	Lemon juice, vinegar		Water		Soap
Scales on hair	Closed				Open
Ease of combing	Silky				Rough

When wet hair is thoroughly dried with a towel, most of the external water will be removed, but not that absorbed by the hair. To remove more, requires a dryer blowing hot air. Excessive drying is not an advantage because if the water content goes below the relative humidity of the surrounding air, it will reabsorb water to reach an equilibrium value of about 10%. On the contrary, very dry hair may become brittle and acquire a static charge making it more difficult to handle.

Research by Unilever in 2004 (Reference 9) confirms that water content in both skin and hair depends strongly on the relative humidity (a well known fact as hair is used in the manufacture of hygrometers for measuring air humidity). In air with a relative humidity below 70%, the water content in hair and the outermost layer of the skin is quite similar, about 10% by weight. Changes in the water or lipid content of skin or hair may affect the feel or look of hair by altering perceptions of dryness, elasticity or brittleness.

A characteristic of hair which should not be overlooked is its rate of growth. Various factors which affect this are discussed elsewhere, such as that growth is fastest in summer and varies with the ethnic group. As a rule, hair grows about 1.25 cm or half an inch per month, so after two months, a permanent wave which had started near the roots would have moved away by one inch. A wave can be rightly called permanent, but the fact remains that it is gradually being pushed out by non-waved hair means that after a few months much of the "permanent wave" may have been removed when the hair is cut.

The Process of Permanent Waving.

It might, at this point, be as well to make quite clear what permanent waving is or was. Many types and makes of machine evolved over these years with continuous feed-back coming from the hairdressers, but the process and machine were basically as follows:

The preliminary phase.
After possibly first tapering the hair to reduce the weight of the ends and make it easier to set, it was shampooed, usually with soap, so it had to be well rinsed because, unlike modern shampoos, it was inherently alkaline.   After drying, the hair was then combed into sections to form up to 22 *locks* (or *mèèches*), so that the base of the lock would look roughly square on the scalp (known as "squaring off" or "sectioning").   The smaller the size of square the closer the eventual winding could start to the scalp.   The experienced stylist would know how to situate these squares and would take into account other factors, such as the position of the parting, or the style which was to be achieved at the end.   In fact, a good stylist would keep in mind the final style he would adopt when choosing the position of the locks.

Each lock was then threaded through a protector, a square or round piece of rubber or felt, which sat on the scalp.   It thus not only maintained the lock of hair together, but also afforded some protection from the heater or any liquid dripping from it, and prevent burning or scalding.

Then the hair either dry or wet according to the method used, was wound on to a former called a *curler*, often made of aluminium for lightness. The choice of curler and the method of winding can be complex and are dealt with at length in Ref. 1, but the first distinction is that winding can start from the end of the lock (or *point-wounding*) or from the root (*root-winding*), being helically wound, when the hair overlaps itself on the curler, or spirally wound when it does not overlap. The distinction is important because with an overlap, the outside tends to get heated more than the inside, particularly near the root where the hair is thicker. It was also believed that point-winding gave greater strength of curl while root-winding gave more perfect waves.

The distinction between point and root winding is most important, because a different type of heater was used in each case; also greater tightness of the curl occurred in a different position in the two cases. For this reason, an early Eugene patent had different heaters for the two ends of the curler. In the case of **root winding**, the hair is simply wound starting from the root, so that the curler stands up from the head and requires a tubular heater, which was the first type used. The hair not only goes around the curler but also travels towards the end of the curler, so it is in the form of a helix, rather like a spiral staircase or the spring in a chest expander. Subtle effects can be achieved by varying the angle at which the hair is applied to the curler, and whether there is any overlap between successive turns of the hair. Overlapping affects the thickness of the layer of the hair, which in turn affects the heating regime required of the heater, particularly near the root of the hair. The most common overlap towards the end of this period was 50%. The position of the element in the heater could be varied so as to give a gradient of temperature from root to point.

In the case of point winding, the end of the lock of hair or mèche could be clipped to the centre of the curler which was then wound towards the root, in the same way as traditional curlers applied by ladies before going to bed. Instead of being helical as with root winding, it was spiral, rather like the spring of a watch. Looked at from this point of view, a root winding is three-dimensional and can be called a curl, while a point winding is two dimensional and should be called a wave, but these terms tend to be used interchangeably.

A point winding as described, was also be called a *croquignole*, and results in the final turns of the winding being thicker than the rest which required a heat gradient giving more heat in the at the roots than at the end. This produced tighter curls at the tip than at the root and gave a different style The heater was of a different design, being more like a bulldog clip which was fastened on to the winding.

The design of the curler and the manner in which the lock was wound (the direction and tension) were often dependent on the preference and experience of the stylist. As the process and styling developed and became more sophisticated, root-winding was used on the top of the head and point winding on the sides, i.e. mixed root and point winding - or mixed winding..

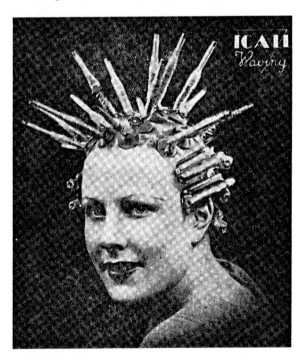

The above picture is a demonstration plate which shows the hair wound on to curlers ready for the sachets and heaters to be applied. The top curlers are root-wound, that is, the winding starts near the root of the hair and proceeds evenly to the top of the curler, where it is held by some device to stop it unwinding. After wrapping the sachet around the curler, the tubular heater is then inserted over the top of the winding. A system combining both types of winding is called mixed winding, and this gave the creative hairdresser greater flexibility in the creation of a style.

The locks at some stage would be treated with a *reagent*, consisting of a chemical dissolved in water, which would prevent the hair from drying out, provide better heat transfer and provide possible reaction with the hair to make it more amenable to curling. The chemical could be something which was mildly alkaline like borax, ammonium carbonate, sodium carbonate or sodium sulphite. Later, for the greater convenience of the hairdresser and to have greater control "sachets" were used consisting of special small pads which would be impregnated with the reagent and wrapped around the winding.

It should now be evident that as compared to the Marcel wave, the geometry of the final curl is different to that obtained by permanent waving. Also, while in Marcel waving only heat was used, the permanent waving process used not only heat, but also steam produced by heating the reagent together with a chemical effect produced by the components of the reagent. Thus, the next stage, in which the lock wound on a curler was inserted into a heater, was referred to as steaming.

The machine stage
Up to this point, there has been no need for a machine, but this is where it came into its own. In its basic form, it consisted of a heavy base on wheels which allowed the machine to be moved easily from customer to customer or out of the way. Because the steaming time rarely exceeded 10 minutes, the time for which the machine was used was considerably less than that of either the preliminary

winding or that of the later setting stage. This meant that one machine could be used for various customers at different stages of the process.

A circular metal canopy was supported by an angled pipe inserted in the base. The pipe had a key which allowed the height of the canopy to be adjusted to the height of the client's head. The angle in the pipe allowed the canopy to be placed centrally over the head of the client.

The chandelier itself was the business end of the machine and its purpose was mainly to take the weight of the heaters, and distribute the electricity to the heaters. Various methods of suspending the heaters were used to facilitate the operation of the machine.

The heaters which were thus suspended were the business end of the machine. The curlers, as prepared in the previous stage, were inserted into the electrically-heated *heaters* which heated or, more correctly in most cases, steamed the hair for a certain time at a certain temperature. These two factors were highly critical and the design of the heaters was of paramount importance. The heaters originally designed by my father were a great advance on anything that already existed, hence their success, and were the subject of much research and patents. The heaters are the objects which, in the photographs of the time, were seen to stick out of the head.

In earlier years, possibly for economic reasons, the number of heaters was only sufficient for doing one half of the head of hair. So the process was carried out in two stages. In the first stage, when the heaters were applied cold, they were left on for ten minutes. They where then transferred to the other half of the head. As they were already hot, they were left on for only left on for six minutes. Times, of course, were dependent on the nature and condition of the hair and the judgement of the hairdresser.

The final phase
After steaming, the heaters were removed and the machine wheeled away. After cooling, the curlers and protectors were removed and

the hair shampooed. The stylist would then get to work to set the hair, using a setting-lotion and hair pins. Finally, the hair held by a hair-net, was dried under a hair dryer.

Everyday technology in the inter-war period

To historians, it may seem that the twenties and thirties - the inter-war or the period of Modernism - is recent history, but to the ordinary person in the street it is a distant and unfamiliar period about which he or she knows little unless they have made a point of learning about it. After all, anyone aged 20 in 1930 would today (and I write in 2006) be 96. Even someone born just after the war would be nearing retirement, and about 16% of the population is 65 years or more of age. Thus, the majority of the population, (including hairdressers) would be unfamiliar with everyday conditions during the interwar period.

Although the beginning of the twentieth century had already taken great strides in technology, most people today would realise that such things as computers and jet aircraft did not exist then. They would probably be less conscious of the absence of some of the most basic items that we take for granted today, which either did not exist at that period or existed only as laboratory curiosities, at least in this country. It might be as illuminating to show what did not exist at a given period as well as explaining what did. Germany, which was already secretly getting itself on a war footing, was seeking new materials, either because of their intrinsic properties, or because they anticipated a shortage of certain raw materials if their sources of supply abroad were curtailed. They were given the name of Ersatz ('substitute') materials a term which in Britain was used as one of contempt for inferior or 'unnatural' products. However, these new materials were not to see general use until after the war, when they had been perfected and were freely available at a reasonable

An advertisement for Bakelite which gives various Icall products as examples of the application of its resins.

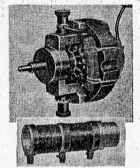
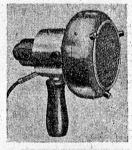
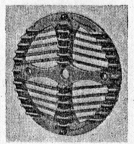
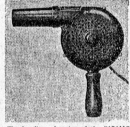
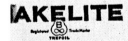

price. The following products are examples of what today may be taken for granted, but that the present day hairdresser may not realise did not exist in those days.

Plastic materials

Plastic materials at the time were in their infancy. Most of those that existed were based on existing natural products or products derived from them. As far back as 1862 Parkes had invented celluloid from cellulose nitrate but it was dangerously inflammable and was replaced by cellulose acetate, but these were mainly used for making films. Cellulose derivatives were also used to make film ('Cellophane') and fibres (Rayon).

However, in 1908, Baekeland invented Bakelite, which is known as a thermo-setting resin because it sets permanently when heated and will no longer flow, so it has to be shaped by compression moulding, while a relatively modern thermo-plastic resin such as polystyrene only becomes solid when it cools and it can therefore be extruded into a mould. A disadvantage of Bakelite is that it tends to be a dark colour, and so only brown and black products could be made. Having said that, it had excellent electric and thermal properties and large, if uncomplicated, mouldings were made for items such wireless cabinets and telephones. I. Calvete Ltd. played a pioneering role in using Bakelite for hairdressing equipment. It was particularly well-suited for making permanent-waving heaters, as they were light and modern-looking and afforded better protection against burns and electric shock. At first, heaters were made for Eugene from cast aluminium, and the individual manufacture of each one must have been expensive. The bakelite replacements must have been much cheaper to make, quite apart from the other advantages it offered. Opposite we can see an advertisement published by Bakelite in 1934 showing the virtues of their new material as first used by Icall. Top left showed a hair dryer motor and components impregnated with resin. Lower left shows the drying element of a dryer secured with resin to the refractory. On the right are two "Icall" hair dryers in which the handle and casing were made from Bakelite Shock-Resisting

Moulding Material. The lower one is of the pistol-type which gives localised drying, while the upper one blows a wider band of air over the whole head.

The cabling for electrical equipment was mainly of rubber, which gave good insulation and flexibility but tended to degrade when exposed to sunlight (specifically, ultra-violet light). Although PVC (polyvinyl chloride) had been known for some time it degraded badly when it was heated. Only in the 30's, when plasticisers became available, could the advantages of PVC be applied to making insulation for cable, but it was not until after the war that it was in domestic use and PVC cables are more or less ubiquitous in the home and elsewhere where electrical devices are used.

Among the plastic materials invented in the thirties, two were of particular significance during the war. Polythene (derived from the chemical name polyethylene) and discovered by ICI was found to have exceptional electrical properties and its use in cables was essential for the development of radar which played such an important role in the Battle of Britain, enabling the fighter pilots, the "Few", to anticipate the arrival of German bombers. A material made from such a cheap raw material excited interested post-war and polythene film soon replaced paper as a packaging material. This in turn led to the carrier bag, the success of which has been so great that it has now become a menace to the environment.

Another ICI product discovered at about the same time was "Perspex", which is a sheet material of high optical clarity achieved by casting between two very large plates of glass which were removed after the material had solidified. It immediately found application in the manufacture of canopies for fighter aircraft and for the gunner and bomb-sight housings of bombers. Important post-war applications which took advantage of its lightness and range of colours were in the manufacture of shop-signs and bath-tubs.

Meanwhile in the United States, Carothers had discovered nylon, the first totally synthetic fibre but which was later also to be used for engineering parts which were lighter than their metallic equivalents and could be manufactured cheaply by injection moulding.

Surfactants

Surfactants (a term originating from "surface-active agents") are so called because they reduce the surface tension of water, in other words, it makes water 'wetter', and therefore wash better. Modern shampoos contain surfactants which make them much more efficient than pre-war shampoos.

The main cleansing agent in a traditional shampoo was soap, a primitive surfactant manufactured from either animal or vegetable fat. Soap is a very old product and it has been suggested that it may have been discovered during the practice of burning sacrificial animals ("burnt offerings") as mentioned in the Bible. The animal to be burnt would be placed above a wood-fire, and the fat from the animal would drop into the fire's ashes which contained potash. Soap is not as efficient as the modern surfactants but one of the main objections to it was that it reacted with lime in hard water, forming a scum which left a film on hair or, if you were having a bath, left an infamous tide-mark which had to be removed afterwards because of its unpleasant appearance. Because some soap was used up in this process, more was used than was strictly necessary for washing and so soap was wasted. Some people were aware that if you used rain-water to wash the hair, less soap was necessary and no scum was formed. Others were lucky and lived in soft-water areas. Proprietary shampoos of the time advised users to wash their hair in two goes. The first removed the dirt but because the soap had been more or less used up by the dirt, did not foam. The second shampoo served to remove any residual dirt but, as most had been removed, this time a foam was formed. The formation of foam had a psychological effect in making the user feel that the hair had been properly washed.

Remember also that in pre-war years, not all houses had laid-on hot-water or fitted baths; showers were relatively rare. When these facilities existed, they were often installed in relatively cold houses and so shampoos and baths were not necessarily an unmitigated pleasure. Whatever the reason, it seems to have been the general custom to have a bath or wash the hair once a week, normally Friday, so that you were nice and clean for the week-end's socialising. Hair would be washed only once a week, - one shampoo manufacturer made a point of this in its advertisements - "Friday night is Amami night".

A common practice at the time was for hairdressers to buy a soft, green soap in drums, and it would be the duty of a junior early each morning to heat some of this up with some water in readiness for the day's work. This may have been a potash soap which was soft and better suited for shampooing. It was probably intended to look like French green soap which was made from olive oil.

Although some of the constituents of modern shampoos were already known, they were not in general use and only became manufactured post-war when there was an upsurge in synthetic products made from petroleum rather than coal. They are generally called surfactants because by reducing the surface tension of water they 'wet' greasy materials more readily. For example, a drop of rain water on glass will tend to remain as a rounded blob, but a surfactant will make it spread over the glass. This effect was demonstrated pre-war, when sensibilities were not so great, by placing a duck in water and adding a small amount of detergent in its vicinity; the water wetted the duck's feathers and the duck gradually sank. Another demonstration of the peculiar properties of such a solution is making bubbles by blowing through a ring which has been dipped in a detergent solution.

Some other primitive surfactants were already in use in pre-war years. An example is what was known as Turkey Red Oil. This was made by a process called sulphation or sulphonation, simply by adding sulphuric acid to castor oil, which turned it a strong red colour – hence the name. It could then be neutralised for use with caustic soda. It had industrial uses such as the demulsification of petroleum which contained water, and as a mordant for dying. It was also used as a primitive shampoo, and for "oil-steaming" as a replacement for purely aqueous reagents.

By February 1935, Icall had introduced "Marsy", which it called a soapless shampoo. Words like synthetic were probably avoided at the time because they were associated with unnatural and inferior substitutes. The product was claimed to shorten steaming times.

It is important to know a little how surfactants work, but I will keep the technical side of this exposition as simple as possible. What we mainly need to know is that there are three types of surfactant: anionic, non-ionic and cationic.

The way an anionic surfactant works is fairly simple. It is obvious to most people that some materials, like salt or sugar, dissolve readily in water while others like oil and grease do not. At one end of the molecules of a surfactant there is a large fatty group which dislikes water (and is called hydrophobic) but is attracted to greasy materials, while the other end of the molecule has a neutralised acid group, which is attracted to water (and is called hydrophilic). The result is a molecule that does not quite know its own mind. What happens is that the ionic part dissolves readily in the water while the fatty end tries to get away. If the molecule reaches the surface, the fatty end tries to get away by sticking out away from the water. This affects the surface properties of the water, and also presents a fatty surface which attracts and holds external fatty materials such as dirt from whatever is being cleaned .

This type of surfactant is called an anionic one, and has totally replaced soap for washing clothes. It is less affected by the hardness of water and does not form a scum. However, it is rather aggressive for use on hair and questions have been asked about its long-term safety when it is used on skin or hair.

A more suitable type of surfactant for washing hair, which is also used for making shower gels, is what is called a non-ionic one, which is therefore neutral, and is a viscous liquid called polyethylene glycol (PEG). It does not contain a fatty group so although it has good wetting characteristics. it is slightly less effective than ionic surfactants and does not foam readily. To enhance the washing power of the shampoo, a certain amount of an anionic surfactant is added, typically sodium laureth sulphate, which is said to be less harmful than some of the earlier anionic surfactants. This also improves foaming which is generally associated with efficiency of washing. Looking at the label on a bottle of shampoo these are shown as the main components, though there is generally a host of others such as perfumes and colouring.

There is a point worth considering regarding the properties of an anionic surfactant used in a shampoo (or for that matter, a shower gel or a bubble-bath product, all of which are similar in principle and composition to a shampoo), is that of the concentration at which it is used. As we have seen, the anionic surfactant acts in two ways: one, it improves the wetting power of water by adding a surface layer of molecules to the water; and it removes grease by combining with it and drawing it into the water. It is difficult to quantify how much surfactant is necessary to do this but we can make an informed guess. To enable the first effect, very little is required and tests have shown that as little as 0.001% is necessary. For the second effect, rather more is required. Excepting cases where large amounts of grease have been added artificially to the hair, it is difficult to imagine the amount of natural grease to be very large - a salt-spoonful? If we reasonably suppose that an equal amount of shampoo would be enough to combine with this, we reach the conclusion that the amounts of detergent used, which are never accurately measured, must be hugely excessive when washing the hair, or for that matter when having a shower or a bath. After all, once you are clean, you are clean and excess surfactant will not make you cleaner. The professional hairdresser might like to consider whether excess amounts of surfactant are being wasted to add more load to the environment.

A third type of surfactant is called cationic. Here, the molecule has the charges the other way round to an anionic one (the fatty group is on the positive rather than the negative end and so acts in a totally way. It is not particularly soluble in water and is not so suitable for washing. The ionic part tends to attach itself to certain types of organic material such as hair, skin, fibres (hence textile conditioners) and paper. and this gives certain useful properties. For example, by attaching itself to the cell walls of bacteria, it acts as a germicide or disinfectant (for example "Savlon"). It also attaches itself to hair, the fatty end sticking out, giving the hair a sheen and soft feel, so cationic surfactants are useful as hair conditioners. They have an added advantage - because they are ionic, they have a modest ability to conduct electricity. Hair which is dried thoroughly in a jet of hot air has a tendency to accumulate static electricity and as every hair acquires the same charge, this to make them separate one from another to give a bulky look, or 'fly-away ends'. A cationic surfactant will lessen this effect.

Because cationic and anionic surfactants are opposites and each neutralises the effect of the other, they cannot easily be combined in a single shampoo and conditioner. One method of creating such a product is to replace the cationic surfactant with a silicone compound which adheres and lubricates the hair so that it can be combed more easily after washing. However, as silicones are strongly water-repellent, it can be difficult to remove them totally in later shampoos and this can cause problems in certain processes where uniform wetting of the hair is essential, such as dying of the hair. Failure to deal with this possibility can result in patchy colouring of the hair, with all its disastrous consequences. On the whole, hair products which contain silicones are not the hairdresser's friend.

Hair conditioners often contain some acid compound which will make the scales of the hair close and make it smoother to comb, after they have been opened by the shampooing process. In olden times, it was known that vinegar and lemon juice has this effect, but modern conditioners tend to contain something like citric acid.

Permanent waving was something carried out only when much of the waved hair had grown out, but before then clients went to the hairdressers for a "shampoo and set". The setting of the damp hair would require something to keep it in place and "setting lotions" were fairly standard. Modern equivalents, such as styling mousses, contain a variety of components, such as water-soluble polymers and cationic/non-ionic surfactants which can look natural without excessive adhesion. In those days, only natural ingredients were available. A common one was gum tragacanth in water, with perhaps a little glycerine for greater flexibility, which was used both for men and women. This also formed the basis, by the addition of coloured pigments, of the so-called 'plastic' style which is mentioned later.

Cold waving

The use of curling 'papers' in Victorian times, and the classical curlers worn over-night to convey some curling to the hair can hardly be called 'permanent'. There may have been some knowledge of chemical ways of waving the hair, but real cold waving is a post-war phenomenon, otherwise there would have been no point in electrical permanent-waving.. My first awareness of cold waving was in about 1950 when a phone call to my father (who was no longer on the development side of hairdressing) from an old friend in Spain enquired about where he could get some thioglycollic acid. He passed the enquiry to me and managed to acquire some and send it, but I was puzzled when told that it was for hairdressing.

It is said that Arnold F. Willatt (presumably in the United States) invented the cold wave in 1938 by applying the knowledge by then acquired of the chemical structure of the hair. A strong reducing agent, ammonium thioglycollate, opens links between the chains of keratin so that in theory, curling the hair in another configuration and restoring the links in the new position, results in a permanent wave. Theoretically, this can be done at room temperature, hence the term 'cold wave', but the time necessary for a successful perm can be reduced by covering with a warm cloth.. A rule of thumb used in chemistry is that an increase of 8 to 10°C in temperature will double the rate of reaction. Thus, covering the hair with a hot towel at 30°C could halve the time required.

I cannot confirm the source from which I learned that cold waving was first used on Afro-American women in the United States. There was a demand for a method which would straighten negroid hair particularly of the extremely curly variety, perhaps to make it less different from caucasian hair and also to make it more manageable or amenable to current styles. Straightening hair is the opposite to waving it, but the heater method available at the time would be unsuitable for straightening hair. Presumably the procedure would be to treat the hair with the ammonium thioglycollate (or other similar compound) and, after a 'soaking' period, combing the hair straight and then neutralising. On the same subject, see the end of Appendix III. I notice that today some hairdressers advertise the straightening of hair by "chemical methods".

Icall Hairdressing Equipment

(a)   The permanent-waving machines.

Permanent-waving machines were made in different formats, one of which was a cabinet used behind or alongside the client, where the heaters were stored and heated, and then applied to the head. However the most used and classic type (see opposite) was a tall support on wheels, which held a "chandelier" which in turn took the weight of the heaters on the head of the seated client. Both Icall and Eugene used this format, although both also made the other type, mainly for use as a portable unit. The earlier models of the classic, tall "chandelier" was the type that was overwhelmingly seen in the majority of salons of the period, and these can be seen in the pictures of Icall exhibition stands in the 20's and 30's, and in many photographs of salons at that time.

The stand or support was fairly universal and had a simple facility for adjusting height and wheels so that the machine could be easily moved to the customer. As one machine would be used sequentially for a number of customers, this was easier than moving a customer to a machine. Besides, when not in use, it could be easily wheeled out of the way. A feature of the stand was that the wheels did not pick up and get tangled with hair which inevitably dropped on the floor of the salon. The heaters also had compensated height adjustment which relieved the weight of the heater regardless of the height of the client.

These heaters were directly connected to the mains while in use. "Safex" heaters were used mainly for root winding, and "Presto" for point winding.

By 1934, Icall had produced its most advanced model, which incorporated all the advances from previous years. It had 16 "Safex" tubular heaters and 4 "Presto" heaters. Below shows an example of a head of hair ready for applying such two types of heaters. The picture opposite shows the ultimate standard Icall machine in which the heaters were directly heated while placed on the head.

This gave the best control of heat. It will be observed that this machine has a device, an Auto-timing Switch, mounted on the supporting tube, which is reproduced opposite. Bari-Woollss made a great point of the importance of accurate timing for permanent waving. The trouble was that the mains voltage used to fluctuate considerably, and affected the temperature of the heater. Thus, by referring to the voltmeter, an adjustment could be made to the steaming time, and this was further corrected by a table on the switch, according to whether the hair was fine, medium or coarse; white or grey; dry or dyed. Having established the correct time, this was set on the auto-timing switch, which automatically switched on the heaters from cold and turned them off at the correct steaming time, at the same time setting off a discrete alarm. Thus, some of the guess-work was removed from the process.

From the start, the technically important part of the machine was the heaters and these were the product of intense research and controversy. Considerable ingenuity was employed in acquiring accurate and uniform temperature control. Some heaters had two windings so that the two sections of hair, one of which might be thicker than the other, could have different heating regimes. Alternatively, the elements could be embedded at a varying depth to produce a gradient of heat. Icall heaters were continually improved since their conception in 1917 until the final versions which were patented in 1934 (Ref. 10). These showed a remarkable sophistication for what outwardly seemed a simple item.

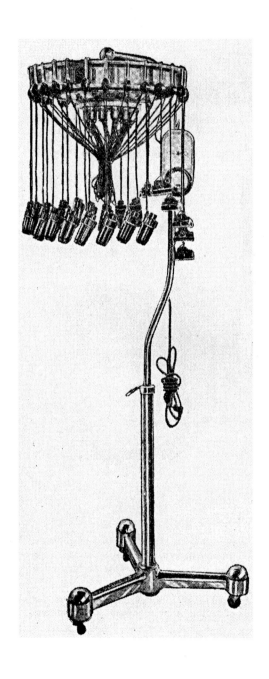

(Left) The ultimate Standard (i.e. "non-wireless") Icall Machine. Variants of this machine could be supplied. Generally, all the heaters were of the traditional "Safex" tubular type, but some or all could be replaced by the "Presto" bulldog type as in this case, so that the sides of the head could be styled differently (called mixed winding). Note also the auto-timing switch (a feature absent in Eugene machines).

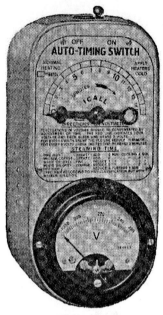

The Automatic Timing Switch which could be supplied with the Standard Machine.

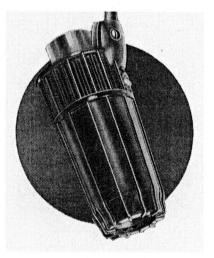

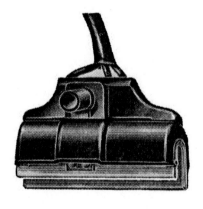

Left: the "Safex" heater   Right: the Presto Heater

(Left) The Auto-Timing switch which took the guess-work out of corrections for varying voltages of the mains supply and different types of hair. The voltage could be read from the dial and a table of hair types just above it gave the following:

Normal Heating Time (Stamped into plate)

Fluctuations of voltage should be compensated by adjustment of time. The red line indicates your voltage and each black line means 2 volts. For every 4 volts above the red line reduce 1 minute. For every 6 volts under the red line increase 2 minutes.

Fine Hair	Greasy	Add 2 min. cooling 4 min.
Medium coarse, Greasy		Add 2 min. cooling 4 min.
White or grey	Coarse	Reduce 2 min., cooling 2 min.
Dry hair		Reduce 4 further minutes

Dyed hair, according to hair classification but with weaker solution.

The heaters below were those developed by Icall using Bakelite which gave a clean appearance and protected the operator's hands from burns. Unfortunately, no information survives on the electrical characteristics of these devices, such as wattage.

An interesting theme that runs through hairdressing literature of the time was safety. This could be sub-divided into chemical safety, physical safety and electrical safety. These were important considerations for hairdressers since accident claims from clients could be costly, quite apart from the loss of custom. Examples of chemical accidents could be burns or allergic reactions from the use of waving chemicals or dyes. Examples of physical accidents could be burns produced by steam emerging on to the scalp from heaters used for waving. However, electrical safety seemed to loom large in the concerns of clients and the psychological appearance of a machine plus the undoubted number of shocks that had occurred because of poor insulation of the heaters. Unsurprisingly, Icall literature constantly refers to the safety of its equipment.

I have no record of electrical incidents with Icall equipment, but there may have been, as insulation in equipment which is in frequent use can get frayed and wet hair and reagents will seek out any flaws in the insulation. To satisfy the demand for greater safety, the Icall-H indirect heating system (sometimes called a wireless system) was developed (see opposite). The heaters are substantially similar to their direct counterparts, but had connector pins which were activated by connecting to sockets in the chandelier. When hot, the heaters were pulled out and applied to the curlers. Superficially, the machines looked the same, but whereas in the original the heaters hung down on a cable, in the H machine cords were used to take the weight of the heaters and contained no conductor.

This machine also had a thermostatic control which was adjusted for the type of hair being waved. The heaters, although similar to the directly heated ones, contained a larger mass of metal, which acted as a heat sink which cooled more slowly. Even so, this method was known as the "falling-heat" method. It was believed to be less demanding because it worked on the basis of the initial temperature being set correctly rather than on length of time of treatment. It was thus independent of variations in the mains voltage. The actual steaming time was between 4 and 8 minutes.

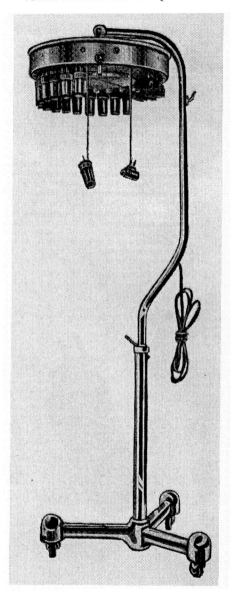

An Icall-H system machine with indirect electrical heating

The Icall-H machine in use. Note the Safex heaters (with root winding) are in the centre of the head, while the Presto heaters (with point winding) are applied to the sides to produce the so-called "mixed winding".

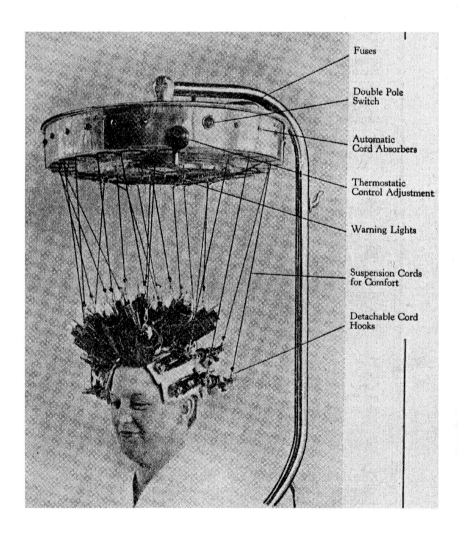

Fuses

Double Pole Switch

Automatic Cord Absorbers

Thermostatic Control Adjustment

Warning Lights

Suspension Cords for Comfort

Detachable Cord Hooks

The Icall-H system was the ultimate machine made by the Company and the last before the fortunes of the Company were overtaken by the war. Ref. 1 describes it as the most radically different machine in Great Britain, in which there was an attempt to overcome all the snags of permanent waving.

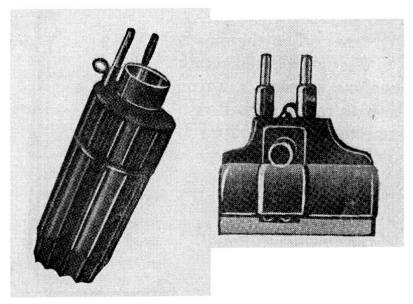

Left: the "Safex-H" heater   Right: the "Presto-H" Heater
These heaters were connected by a cord (a plain string which took the weight) to the chandelier where they were plugged in at mains voltage to heat up. They were then pulled out and thus disconnected before being applied.

"Safex-H" heaters were used for root winding, and "Presto-H" for point winding. Claims for the machine were that it was safe (there were no electric wires direct to the head); it used what was called True Falling Heat, with thermostatic control; and required only one type of reagent of low strength with resultant low running costs and minimum damage to the hair.

(b) The dryers

Hardly any visit to a hairdresser avoids the need for hair to be wetted in some way or other and hence dried before the lady can leave the salon. Also, a number of hairdressing processes require the hair to be clean but dry; hair already saturated with water will not readily absorb solutions of chemicals for say, waving or dyeing, and what does enter the hair will be diluted by the water already in it. So it goes without saying that hair should be dried with a jet of dry, preferably hot, air to remove not just the surface moisture but also some of that that has penetrated the hair. The principle used is that air with less than 100% relative humidity will absorb water, and heating the air makes it not only more comfortable but reduces the relative humidity considerably.

The electric hairdryer must have been accepted immediately as an invaluable tool, even before permanent-waving became established. Certainly, my father was repairing and, soon after, manufacturing hairdryers after 1917. These were of the handheld type. The one on the left (page opposite), which can be described as a pistol dryer, can be seen as the precursor of present day dryers, except that it is made of different materials. The main casing was of aluminium, but the large motor made it a heavy article to hold. The switch was a ceramic rotary one and the handle was of painted wood. The flexible cable was of rubber insulation covered with woven cotton. The hand-held dryer on the right (the "Ultra"), was developed later as a means of drying the whole head with a wider but less intense jet of air. It was claimed to produce a very large volume of hot air, not approached by any other hand dryer, was the only alternative to helmets (which then did not exist) and was quicker than other dryers using a trunk.

Early exhibition photographs showed that a simple solution not only to the weight problem, but also that of taking up an assistant for the drying process was a stand to which the dryer could be attached. However, there was an obvious need for something more suited for professional work and the mounting of the motor and air impeller on

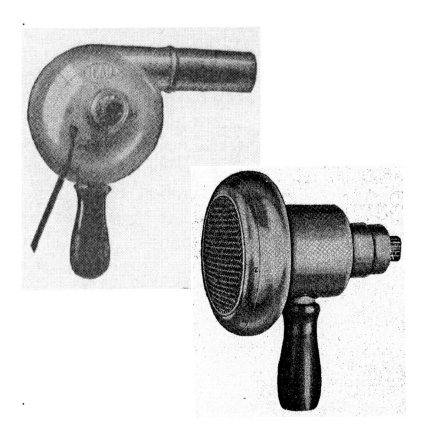

a mobile stand was an obvious step. However, the idea of directing the flow of air by hand persisted , and to do this, flexible trunking was connected to the motor unit, so that the assistant still had to hold the trunking and direct the flow of air.

No account would be complete without the earliest model of a pedestal dryer that I have been able to find which was called - for obvious reasons - the "Non-Electric Pedestal Hairdryer for use where no current is available". It was described as follows (see picture):

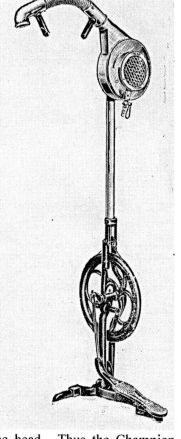

"This Hairdryer has a foot motor or treadle to produce the power, which by means of a concealed belt, rotates the fan inside the drum.

Requires very little effort to maintain a high speed and gives off a substantial draught. It is adjustable to any angle and the hot air is obtained by a gas burner. Very efficient and of pleasing appearance. All the fittings above the fly-wheel are nickel plated."

A small leap of the imagination suggested rigid trunking which just blew the air onto the top of the head. Thus the Champion Pedestal dryer was born (see opposite, left), and although it was designed for electrical use, a gas-heated version was also made. Because the trunking took up some room, it was hinged in the middle so that it could be folded when not in use. This version came out in about 1925.

The Champion was also advertised for medical and other uses: "The temperature of the air at the nozzle is raised above 300 degrees and drops as the distance increases; the pressure of the air is so great that

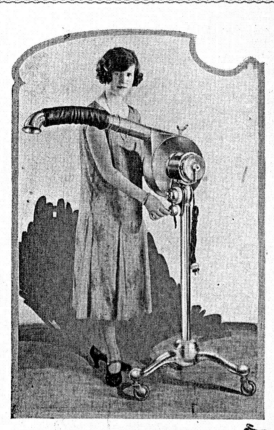

The Champion Pedestal Hair Dryer

This machine is of irreproachable quality, and is specially recommended for use in busy establishments where time is valuable. It can be set to work instantly, and the amount of air required is easily regulated by a three speed controlling switch with which the motor is provided.

Hot air is obtained either by gas or electricity, in the case of the former the gas burner can be regulated by two independent taps; if the air is to be heated by electricity, a special switching arrangement prevents the heating element being put into operation without the motor being also in circuit. This device—exclusive to the "Champion"—renders the heating element entirely fool-proof.

The Motor is very powerful and runs silently for long periods without overheating. The drum, fan and

flexible tube are highly finished and very substantial, and all the fittings are nickel plated. The base is mounted on special large castors and is also nickel plated, under the switch is a swivel on which the whole of the top part swings easily in any direction. The drum rotates on the side, thus enabling the nozzle to be raised or lowered, and by means of a coupling device it can be turned to any desired position.

The Champion Pedestal Dryer is the result of many years experience in the construction of Electrical Hairdressing apparatus of this kind—it will give a lifetime of satisfactory service.

Specify voltage and current when ordering, if alternating current, the number of cycles must be mentioned. Also state whether heated by gas or electricity.

WEIGHT	CODE WORD
69 lbs.	"Champion"

PRICE. £18 18 0 D.C.   £19 19 0 A.C.

it produces the sensation of massage when it comes into contact with bare flesh. As used by the medical profession it is of great value in various diseases and is convenient for drying infectious and discharging wounds. Hairdryers are very efficient for warming beds, linen and towels, drying photographic plates and other purposes."

A less bulky equivalent of the Champion pedestal dryer was produced for smaller salons in about 1929, called the Championette, which allowed the fitting of various drying fittings. However it was mainly designed for a new Icall fitting called the Adjusto (see below), consisting of three sets of piping which could be adjusted to the head of the client. The piping contained holes through which the hot air emerged on to the head, and did not require the constant attendance of an assistant to dry the hair, in fact it could be the precursor of the 'helmet' type of dryer (see opposite). Although an alternative flexible trunk could still be supplied for the traditionalist (see below the Adjusto), it was the first step taken by Icall towards towards the ubiquitous hood or canopy hair dryer of today.

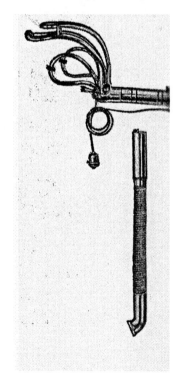

The next stage in the development of the hair dryer was to produce a model which did not require an assistant to hold or direct the trunking. This was the classic hood dryer, still in use today. Its origins are obscure, it may have crossed the Atlantic from the U.S., but in Britain the iniative was taken by a company not involved in hairdressing called Marchant Hills, with a model called the "Sphinx", but the company went bankrupt. Eugene experimented with an all-metal model in the U.S. which was not too successful in Britain. Icall's first model in the field, in the early 1930's and based on the Sphinx, was called the "Quix" dryer as shown by the following advertisement.

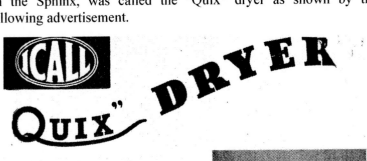

MORE AIR!
MORE DRYING POWER!

WITH THE FAST-DRYING "QUIX"
THE OUTSTANDING SUCCESS
HAIR DRYERS . . .

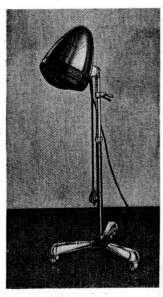

- Fitted with a silent, self-lubricating motor, totally enclosed in a dust-proof casing.

- Positive re-circulation has eliminated all possibility of cold spots, without affecting the tremendous output of the Dryer, or the degree of comfort necessary to the customer.

- The controlling switch is fully protected with thick rubber, eliminating every possibility of risk when handled by the customer.

- The chromium plated hood is provided with compensated balancing mechanism for easy adjustment to the head ; the handsome stand has one hand " fool-proof " height adjustment lever, whilst the base is fitted with hairproof castors.

- All components are robustly made, and the working parts have been so designed that maintenance costs will be found negligible.

PRICE **16** GNS.

Or Hire Purchase Terms: Deposit £2.10.0 and 12 Monthly Payments of 25/-.

CALVETE LTD. ICALL WORKS. NORTH ST. CLAPHAM. SW4
DEMONSTRATIONS & SHOWROOM · 52 DEAN ST. LONDON. W.I.

The "Quix" dryer used a similar base to that used for the permanent waving machines, but also had a spring-loaded hood which was easily adjusted with one hand by releasing the lever. The switch dangled from the hood so that the client could exercise some control if the heat became uncomfortable. It claimed some re-circulation of the heated air which must have increased its efficiency.

However, this was a precursor of the "Perfex" hairdryer, the most sophisticated and the last designed by Icall, which was described as a suction dryer. All other dryers worked on the simple principal of a motor which turned a fan which sucked in air and then blew it through a heated element and thence onto the client's hair. In most cases, the air was not re-circulated.

At this distance in time, it is not entirely clear why the "Perfex" was called a suction dryer. The dryer itself was of an elegant and original design and had an internal casing of Bakelite which came into contact with the head. The casing contained an arrangement of holes which contributed to the re-circulation of air. The impression I have is that instead of sucking air from the back and pushing it out of the front as was the usual case, a relatively small amount of air was sucked in from the front taken to a chamber behind the hood, where it was heated and circulated by means of the Bakelite lining. An amount of air equivalent to that introduced at the front would be expelled at the back. Apart from a greater efficiency, such an arrangement would do away with the discomfort of hot air blowing over the face of the client.

Some of the claims made for the "Perfex" were: "The penetrating air action caused by the special re-circulating process of the apparatus prevents the harsh baking effect, and the hair is dried in a very short time. Cold spots are entirely eliminated by a perfect and logical distribution of the hot air." "The interior of the hood which comes into contact with the head consists of a large Bakelite moulding, which ensures safety to the customer from electric shock." "The head is highly finished in cellulose and is available in two colours: Olive Green and Black." "This time-saver does the work at very low operating costs, in fact, less than a hand dryer. " In spite of the claims, the "Perfex" was sold at the same price as the "Quix". 16 guineas was equivalent to £16.80, a considerable sum in those days.

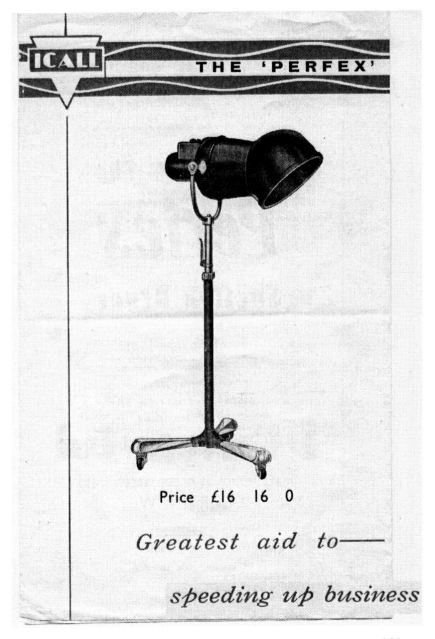

ICALL

THE 'PERFEX'

Price £16 16 0

Greatest aid to——

speeding up business

(Opposite) The I. Calvete stand at the British Industries Fair of 1934. This picture is of interest because it shows the full range of dryers ever made by the company - presumably there was still a market for the earlier models. From the left, we can see the two hand models, the pistol type being mounted on a stand; At the back, there is an unknown canopy dryer (a prototype?), a "Championette" fitted with a trunk, and a very long trunk to the right of it , and then a "Champion" with a folded trunk; at the front, there are two "Perfex" models, the one on the left showing a clear view of the interior with its sophisticated air circulation system; at the very right, there is a hand-dryer with a Bakelite case. Between the two "Perfex" models, there is an "Ajusto" model. By 1936, the hairdressing shows concentrated on the "Quix" and "Perfex" for use by professional hairdressers.

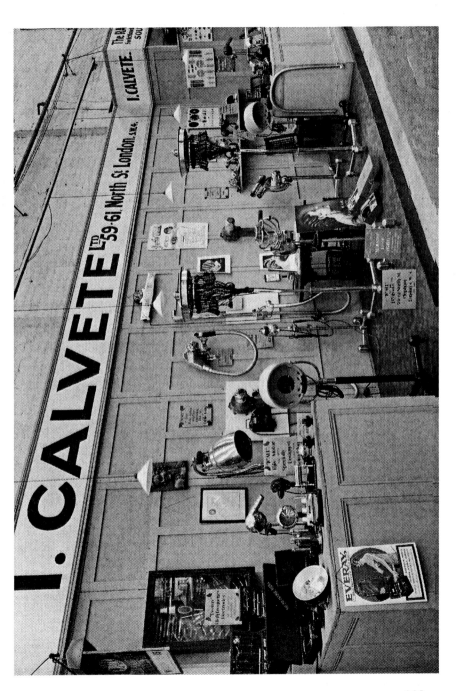

(c) The Curlers

The curlers may seem the humblest of components but they were given great importance both by the manufacturers of systems and hairdressers, mainly because the former believed they affected results and the latter was because they were the ones who had the trouble to wind wet hair on to them. Therefore, anything that simplified and speeded up the process was desirable. Attempts were made to mechanise the winding process, but it was generally accepted that hand winding was the best.

Root winding

In both types of winding, some protection was necessary for the scalp from the heat of the heater and, to some extent, from the reagent that was applied to the hair. This protection generally took the form of a circular or square piece of rubber or felt with a hole through which the hair was threaded with a hook or, preferably, the hair was passed through a slot cut from the hole to the edge. Originally, the hair was then wound on to a curler and held at the hair end with a clip. Reagent or a moistened sachet was then applied, and the whole might be covered with metal foil to reduce evaporation. The curlers would then lie against the head until inserted in the heater. In the 30s, Icall and others introduced curlers with a clip fixed at the bottom end of the curler, so that the latter would stick out. This made it easier for a single person to wind the hair

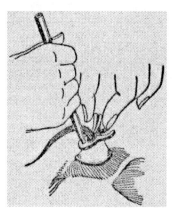

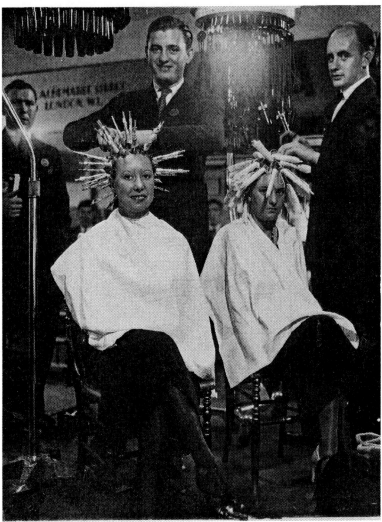

1932 Exhibition at Olympia, London. An interesting comparison of the two ways of root winding. The right-hand one is the traditional method where the curlers just lie on the head until inserted in the heaters. The left-hand one has the curlers fixed and are wrapped in foil, so that they stuck out, making it easier for one person to wind them and to apply the heaters. This method came from Goumy in Paris. Note that 100% root-winding was used in both cases. The gentleman on the right was an Icall demonstrator.

Point winding

Where root and point winding were used together (mixed winding) point winding was generally limited to the sides of the head. While in root winding, the curler remained more or less stationary and the hair was wound round the curler, in point winding , the point was caught up on the curler and wound on in an action similar to that of rolling a cigarette.

First, however, the hair was threaded through a rectangular pad, similar in principle to the that used in root-winding, and the hair clamped with a small clamp. When the hair had been wound on to the curler, the curler was clipped into the clamp in such a way as to maximise the tension of the hair. The hair was then treated with reagent or covered with a sachet and/or metal foil in the same way as for root-winding.

Below: Icall point-winding curlers

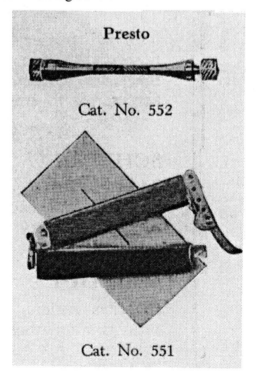

Presto

Cat. No. 552

Cat. No. 551

(d) The sachets

It has been seen that permanent waving is achieved by steam in the presence of certain chemicals to assist in the reformation of the hair structure, because in this way better waving is obtained with less damage to the hair. The chemical was in the form of aqueous solutions ("reagents") but so-called oil was sometimes recommended in the case of fragile hair or to prevent the yellowing of white hair. Icall sold its own reagents (as did other manufacturers) and so did hairdressing wholesalers.

The presence of water played three important roles in the hairdressing process. First, it transmitted heat efficiently from the heater to the hair. Second, together with any chemicals it contained, it altered the structure of the hair so it adopted the shape of the winding into which it had been made. The third reason is important but not so immediately obvious. An advantage over Marcel waving was that there was less risk of overheating and thus damaging the hair. This is only because while there is water present the temperature cannot go much above the boiling point of water, i.e. 100°C. The more the temperature is above this, the more water will evaporate to keep it at this temperature. Generally, the water applied as reagent directly on the hair was not enough to avoid the hair drying our before the process ended. So, from the earliest days something like a wet pad was wrapped round the curler so that there would be more water present. This could be done in root winding by using what was called a "sachet" which was wetted before wrapping round the curler.

I believe the originator of the sachet was a man called Charles Kropacsy, a first-line hairdresser and collaborator of Eugene, who regularly contributed to the Hairdressers' Weekly journal. It may have been a reaction to the original, cumbersome, Nessler technique in which cardboard tubes were immersed in a bucket of reagent before inserting them over the curlers.

The word "sachet" is not really a good term for what it portrayed but was the term which was universally used by the trade at the time for a certain permanent waving requirement. Even then, as now, sachet meant a small, sealed rectangular package which would contain a liquid or a powder, for example shampoo. In this context, however, it took the form shown in the drawing. The main body of the sachet B was a piece of vegetable parchment paper which carried the name of the maker. Parchment paper was made by passing good quality paper through sulphuric acid which gave it a gelatinous consistency; it was then washed to remove the acid and dried producing a sheet rather like parchment. Because it tended to be brittle, a small amount of glycerine was added to plasticise it and a small amount of blue dye to conceal the the yellow colouration (compare this with a blue rinse to conceal the yellowness of grey hair). The product is a tough water- and steam-resistant film (nothing like grease paper which is just paper impregnated with paraffin wax).

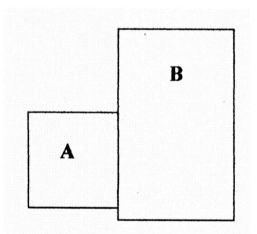

Section A enclosed a felt pad, impregnated with the right chemicals. Access of water was possible through small punched holes in the paper or by placing a small gauze window over the pad. (Goumy of Paris took this to its logical and simple conclusion and just fixed a felt pad to the edge of the paper.) The moistened section A was then wrapped round the root end of hair followed by section B so that the lock of hair was held in a tube. Goumy also conceived the idea of improving the seal by wrapping a piece of aluminium foil round the paper, which reduced steam loss, gave good heat conductivity and could be used to stand the curler vertically making it easy to add the heater.

The sachet could thus be a labour-saving device which speeded up a lengthy part of the operation. From the manufacturer's point of view, it was a useful source of continuous income as up to 36 sachets could be used per customer and they were not supposed to be reusable. (A modern equivalent which comes to mind is the computer printer which may not be expensive, but which uses ink cartridges which have to be continuously replaced as the ink is used up.)

It was a complementary but continuous source of profit compared to the 'one-off' nature of the sale of machines. Consequently in the thirties, something of a "sachet war" started to capture the loyalty and money of hairdressers. Eugene was charging one guinea (£ 1.05) for a gross box of sachets, Icall charged 8/6 (£ 0.43).and Osborne & Garret 4/6 (£ 0.23). As can be seen, it could be a nice little earner.

The price of Icall sachets was 8/6 (43p) a gross. If 24 were used on a head, this would cost 7p, which would be about £2.70 in today's money. A fashionable hairdresser might not think this important, but one with a cost-conscious clientele might think this excessive. They would probably buy the cheapest reagent in bulk and re-use the sachets several times. However, Eugene charged 21/-, that is one guinea per gross. (For those unfamiliar with pre-decimal currency, a guinea was one pound and one shilling, a relic of the days when some gold coins contained more gold than others. The guinea, apart from being a trick to charge 5% more than what appeared to be the value in pounds, was also a snobbish way of making a product appear more classy than it really was. A shop with a range of products might charge pounds for the cheaper ones and guineas for the more expensive ones. Professional people, like solicitors and doctors, would often charge in guineas. As far as I know, today the only things priced in guineas are race horses and pictures.)

However, if you wanted the prestige of advertising yourself as a Eugene hairdressers, you had to use their sachets. They were also wise to tricks like using Eugene sachets at the front of the head and cheaper ones behind. Sachets therefore became an important source of income, perhaps greater than the sale of the equipment that used them.

The advertisement opposite for Express sachets appeared in the HJ dated the 1st April 1939 and is particularly poignant because it appeared the day after my father resigned from the company and is the last known Icall advertisement I have found associated with the original company.

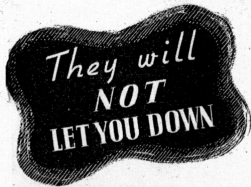
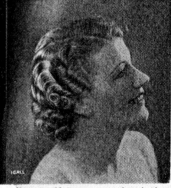
111

The Competition

A t this distance in time, I see the development of permanent-waving as originating mainly from three individuals, from Nessler - for having the idea, from Eugene - for publicising it, and from Calvete for the technical development. But of course there were also other innovators and imitators who entered the field, some of which introduced interesting and useful ideas. The Icall models have been described

Nestlé*
Karl Nessler is generally credited with patenting an invention in 1909 for electrical permanent waving to supersede attempts to wave by winding hair on to a curler and steaming it with hot irons, or waving it loose as in Marcel waving. In 1914 he developed a tubular heater on which future heaters would be loosely based. It was designed to deal with the long hair of the time and consisted of a cylindrical electric heater which allowed the ends of the hair to remain outside. The shorter hair which became acceptable and fashionable after the First World War allowed the development of smaller and more efficient heaters, and Nestlé developed three systems:

The Radione System, in which the hair is wound dry and inserted into hollow cellophane tubes with a moistened, absorbent paper tube which contained the reagent. The ends of the tube were sealed with clips and the tube inserted in the heater. Care had to be taken to avoid scalding, but the system was said to produce waves of beautiful softness.

*The man was called Nessler, but the Company and its products were called Nestlé.

The Oleum System was a departure from Nessler's earlier methods in that it was a wet-wound system using a reagent which contained a certain amount of oil. The reagent was present in fabric strips which were moistened and wrapped round hair winding. The heater was designed to give perfect centering of the winding but seems rather cumbersome.
The Triumph System was a mixed winding system introduced when this became the most versatile system of working

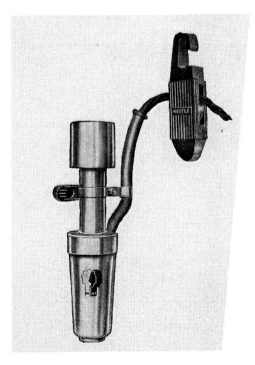

The Nestlé oleum heater

Eugene

The Eugene system came into existence in 1917 and was based on a double-winding of the element so that the root end of the hair could be heated more than the rest. This was desirable because the hair is coarser and more abundant near the roots. However, the idea was covered by Nestlé's patents. To quote Ref. 1 "Then it was that I. Calvete and Eugene performed a miracle almost in a night. A piece of ingenious invention was produced which converted Eugene's curler into the two-way perfection which is now known all over the world".

Page 26 shows the prototypes of the curlers which clearly show the two windings. Eugene probably introduced the idea of a sachet to improve the steam nearer the root and gave greater durability of the wave.

Macdonald.

In the early days of permanent-waving, because of the imperfect apparatus and reagents, the amount of steam available for the process, was limited, and an inexperienced operator could damage the hair by overheating. Macdonald attempted to circumvent this by using steam both to heat the hair and to keep it moist. In the first model, the steam came from a small boiler mounted on the stand (see opposite) but this resulted in unequal heating so later models had 24 small kettles located round the crown of the machine, the steam being led by rubber tubes to the steam jackets on the hair. Because the reagent was volatile (probably some form of ammonia, which could be inserted in the kettles or as a solid pastille inserted inside the jacket), the hair was treated with almost pure steam and the hair did not dry out. Provision had to be made to collect the condensation which formed in the curler.

Macdonald Systems recommended two-handed winding, in which an assistant held the curler firmly pressed against a finger placed upon the rubber protector (which prevents steam reaching the scalp) while the operator wound with two hands, taking the mesh to be wound alternately in each hand. This enables very tight winding, though this is not strictly necessary for good waving.

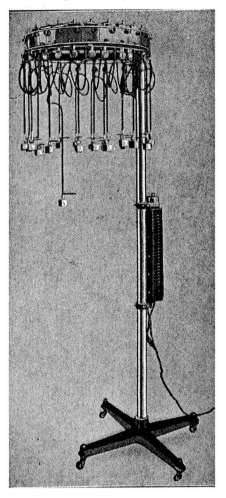

Early Macdonald model with the kettle on the upright of the stand. The cables and heaters of the conventional machine are replaced by rubber tubing and connectors for the jackets, so there is no direct electrical connection.

Macdonald Steam Jackets which were connected to the boiler with rubber tubing by means of the connectors hanging down . (These are not heaters). Considerable loss of heat took place and so the distance was shortened by placing individual kettles on the chandelier.

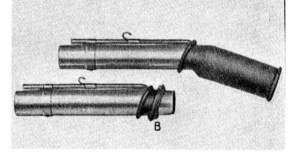

Macdonald was sponsored and financed by Osborne and Garrett, the wholesalers. Macdonald had a fair success at hairdressing competitions because the low temperature produced soft, natural-looking waves, but it was not a marketing success because clients preferred a quicker and more pronounced type of wave.

Macdonald had a claim to fame in 1936, because it was chosen for use in the hairdressing salon of the "Queen Mary" which was launched about this time for the prestigious Southampton to New York sea-crossing. The reason for the choice may have been that Osborne and Garret had succeeded in getting the contract for the installation of the gentlemen's and ladies' hairdressing salons on the vessel and they naturally sponsored Macdonald.

Macdonald was one of the few firms to continue advertising in the HJ throughout the war.

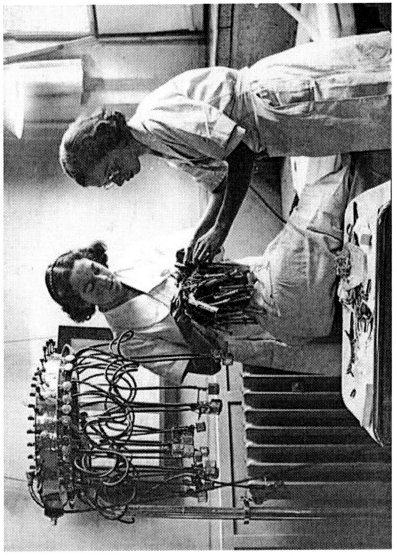

Photograph dated c.1930 showing women's hairdressing class: two students preparing client for permanent wave treatment. (Courtesy London College of Fashion).This is the later model of the Macdonald with small kettles installed in the chandelier, above the client's head.

Gallia

J. Metelski, the man behind the Gallia name, is credited with inventing the technique of moistening the hair with reagent before winding - hitherto it had always been wound dry, presumably deriving from the Marcel method. After winding, the wet hair was only protected in the heater by a wrapping of paper or other material. Wet-winding produced much better results, but made the winding more difficult. The meshes of hair have to be continually combed in order to ensure flat, tight winding. Metelski was also credited with oil processing and Gallia may have been first firm to introduce mix winding. The Gallia machine seems to have evolved from the Nessler machine, and a later machine, the Gallia-Rollair, was produced later for mixed-winding. The claim made for this system was that it was very fast. The Gallia show-room was located in Albemarle Street.

Superma

The man behind the Superma Systema was a Mr Sartory. It was a machineless system, that is, it did not use electric heaters. The method employed so-called cassettes of absorbent cellulose which contained an unspecified chemical which reacted with water when wetted, increasing the temperature and emitting steam. There was no outer casing used, although at some stage, metal foil was added to the outside of the cassette. As the operating conditions were fixed and did not allow variations in time or temperature, the process was controlled by varying the amount of reagent according to the texture of the hair. The method appeared to be in great vogue on the Continent and in North America.

Gensurco (see opposite) This name derives from the General Surgical Company which had considerable experience in the manufacture of permanent-waving machines, although they tended to follow existing practice. Their machines came with metal liners for the heaters (which had an outward similarity to the Eugene ones) to reduce the internal diameter and make them more suitable for oil permanent waving. The impression given by the machine was that it was built down to a price, and it was sold direct to hairdressers at 21 guineas (£22.05) with 12 heaters and all accessories. It was claimed that one client per month paid off your instalment. It was claimed to be the "Queen of P.W. Machines".

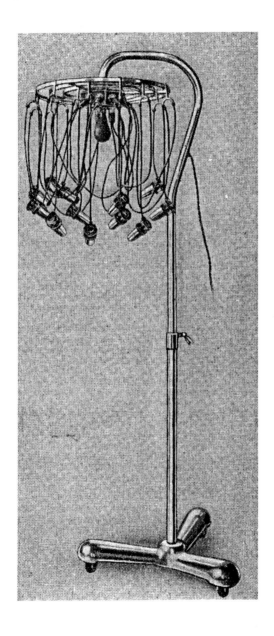

Wella-Rapid
The Wella machine was of German origin which worked as an all-croquignole system. An important feature of the machine was that it reduced the voltage of the system to a safe level (a technique later adopted by Eugene). There seemed some risk of inadequate heating as an external heater was also provided. it did away with the classic chandelier so there was no mechanism to support the weight of the heaters. On the other hand, the machine was undoubtedly elegant and would not look out of place in a modern establishment.

Frigidine
Originally, heaters were generally made with a metallic casing the thermal radiation from which could cause considerable discomfort, and in some cases, burn to the client and to the operator as well. The Frigidine System was conventional except that it used bakelite cases like the Icall ones, to reduce the heat radiated by the heater, and of course they offered electrical insulation as well thermal insulation. It was one of the few machines at the time to incorporate a timing-mechanism.

Madison PSF and Cadex were cabinet machines and might have been preferred by ladies of a nervous disposition. However, the absence of a chandelier meant there was nothing to take the weight of the heaters or to prevent them drooping. The Belleville-Lister was a portable machine useful for the hairdresser who visited the customer. Both Eugene and Icall made such machines.

Vapeur Marcel, a French steam system based on principles similar to the Macdonald one. It is mentioned here because Eugene in later years showed an interest in the method which in any case was overtaken by events.

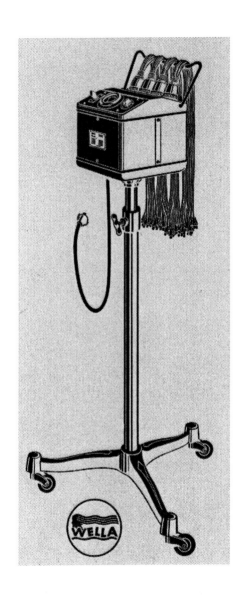

The Wella-Rapid Machine

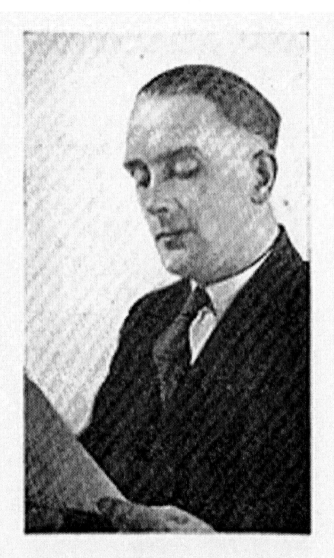

Mr. J. BARI-WOOLLSS

J. Bari-Woollss

This narrative would hardly be complete without mentioning J. Bari-Woollss, a professional chemist, who was employed by my father from about 1931. This perhaps was the first serious attempt to introduce some science into hairdressing processes, as much of what had preceded was empirical. From his knowledge of hair and the experience while working with I. Calvete Ltd., he was able to publish a book, "The Manual of the Permanent Waver", published in 1934 by the Westminster City Publishing Company, which attempted to bring a bit of logic to the differing points of view on how permanent-waving was best carried out. By then, much was already known of the chemistry of hair but this had not been applied to permanent waving. He went to great lengths on the technology of winding hair, but he also investigates some of the chemistry of hair. The combination of an unusual style and unfamiliar science may have made this a bit difficult for a hairdresser to understand, but it had the merit of comparing the different processes and manufacturers. He was a frequent contributor to the Hairdressers' Weekly Journal where he published his findings and after leaving I. Calvete Ltd., he became editor of, and contributor to, a rather magnificent book "The Art and Craft of Hairdressing" published just before the war.

It was a second edition of the book first published in 1931, revised in view of the great strides made since then, but the original author and editor, G. A. Foan, had died before completing the revision of the second edition. It is a rich source of hairdressing history and makes considerable reference to the products of I. Calvete Ltd. (Ref. 2)

The Icall catalogue for 1934 contained the following

"Our Research Department advises the hairdresser on all trichological problems; it carries out continuous research into the subject of hair and permanent waving besides carrying out pure research.

Our Director of Research is Mr. J. Bari-Woollss. He is noted for having in 1931 brought before the trade a new revolutionary theory of permanent waving based upon a close study of contemporary pure research in fibre physics and protein chemistry. His practical and scientific knowledge of the subject of permanent waving has been proven to be authoritative over a period of many years from his contribution to trade literature. His work along these lines has created a powerful impetus in the study of hair theory."

Bari-Woollss credits Astbury and Woods, who were textile researchers, of Leeds University with the discovery that hair is mainly composed of keratin, a protein which also occurs in nails and skin. Long chains of keratin are aligned with the main direction of the hair. These chains are linked one to another with links which may be broken by heat which facilitates waving.

However he was not only a theorist but was deeply conscious of the practical problems of hairdressers. This he expresses in a somewhat unusual style. The following is an interesting example, which is also a reflection on the social attitudes of the time. I can only guess that some of the women mentioned must be middle-class, single and led a busy social life:

"I now wish to deal with a branch of permanent waving which, although not the highest, is nevertheless fairly general. I refer to what might be termed half-perms and repairs.

When hairdressers congregate and discuss permanent waving, we can divide them usually into two camps. The first camp, and, in my opinion, the most highly cultured camp, regards permanent waving from the point of view of art. These workers will not tackle a job unless they can see at the finish a beautiful head of hair effectively dressed and presenting a spectacle to the eye which, to say the least of it, is comparable with the effects that can be obtained upon a head of naturally wavy hair. The second group of hairdressers is by far the majority. They are merely concerned in the long run with the obtaining of results which will satisfy the customer regardless of any artistic tenets, and despite any peculiar ideas of their own as to what constitutes or not a beautiful permanent wave. As I have said, they are the backbone, the rank and file of the Hairdressing Trade, and most of my sympathies are with them. These are the people who have to turn out a commodity of practical standard value. Provided that the hair of their customers will set up into deep waves and tight curls, the waves being arranged more or less concentrically around the parting, they are satisfied.

Moreover, these sets must stand up against at least two weeks' wear and tear of the kind which their customers have to endure. Their clients are not women who can step out of their hairdressers' cubicles into their car only to go straight from there to the social function for which they have had their hair specially set. No, they are women who have to rise early in the morning, hurriedly take their bath, hastily dress their hair, precipitately catch the 8.20 to town, and there do eight to ten hours' hard work. When they leave the office or works they must be able to dash off to their homes with a minimum of time wasted upon a tousled coiffure. They have no time, therefore, for anything in the way of fancy dressings, for the dressings have to be suitable for outdoor wear, the office, the tennis court, and the theatre.

This huge number of women are the bread and butter of the Hairdressing Trade. And for obvious reasons they cannot afford to spend much money upon highly elaborate work. A permanent waving system, or a permanent waver who cannot produce the hard, commercial wave which these millions of women require is not worthy of the name. I have in mind a well-known system, which, while it is capable of producing some of the most artistic results the

Trade has ever seen, is yet often unable to produce in the hands of the average assistant the durability which is so much desired.

Among these customers are numbers who are not prepared to pay for a complete perm when their old one has nearly grown out. They ask you to re-perm the sides, or to put a line of curlers along the parting, or to re-wave the undergrowth at the neck in the case of long bobs. All these are jobs which the unhappy suburban hairdressers are expected to undertake. And indeed if one refuses to carry out such a job, there are always competitors who will find some way to satisfy such demands. We must, therefore, decide what can be done in the way of such patchwork jobs.

A great deal depends upon the psychology of the customer, for sometimes a little judicious explanation will convince her that such work is a compromise which contains all the vices of permanent waving and few, if any, of the virtues. To take, for example, the case of a line of curlers down the parting, this is often asked for when the first wave has grown down to the level of the eye. The customer is perfectly satisfied that by running a line of curlers along the parting she can hide the age of her perm without going to the expense of a complete re-wave."

The reagents that were used to complement the waving process seem to have been chosen by trial and error. Until the time of Bari-Woolls, an alkaline reagent seemed to be favoured, starting with the excessively alkaline caustic soda used by Nessler, to milder materials such as borax. Ammonia became a preferred material because it did not leave a residue. About the time of Bari-Woolls, and he may have been the instigator, reducing agents were found to be more effective. In chemistry, a reducing agent is the opposite of an oxidising agent, that is, it either removes oxygen or adds hydrogen. The various types of sulphite that exist are reducing agents and enable the operator to cut down the steaming temperature or reduce the steaming time. A particularly powerful reducing agent is thioglycollic acid which eventually would lead to cold waving.

126

I know about the sulphites because when Bari-Woollss departed, my father brought all his chemicals home, where I added them to my chemistry set, including materials such as sodium sulphite, sodium bisulphite and sodium metabisulphite. Also some chemistry books which instilled in me the desire to become a chemist.

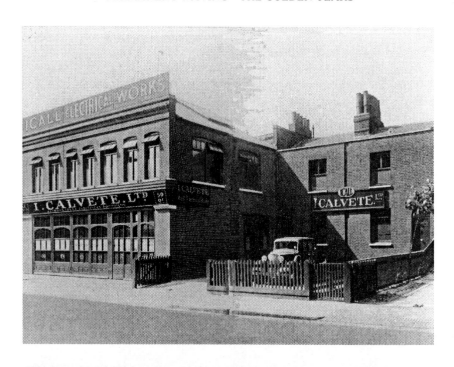

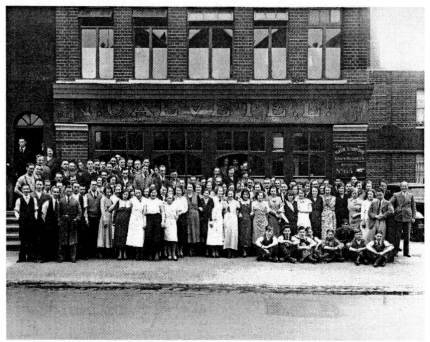

The Clapham Factory and Staff Events

The picture left/top shows the factory at 59 North Street, Clapham, London SW4. When compared with the photograph below, it can be seen to have been modified for publication purposes, by an artist's addition of another section.

The lower photograph taken in 1934 shows the factory staff numbering some 110 persons, which did not include staff in the show-room in London and salesmen and demonstrators on the road. Some of the staff had come from the previous premises in Little St. Andrew Street, and some of the girls travelled every day from Camden town where some manufacturing had taken place. My father is on the extreme right.

The fate of the premises is unclear. When my father left in 1939, Eugene may have started to transfer production in North London, but in any case, most such premises were immediately converted to war production and little in the way of luxury items would have been produced.

A visit today to the site shows that everything to the right of No. 57, that is from where the man is standing in the doorway at the extreme left, has disappeared and has been replaced by post-war dwellings. The likely explanation is that in October 1940, the German blitzkrieg was unleashed on London and this area was heavily bombed, because Clapham Junction was only one mile to the West, and was an important strategic target.

The following pages show some views of the inside of the factory. which are fairly typical of factories of the period.

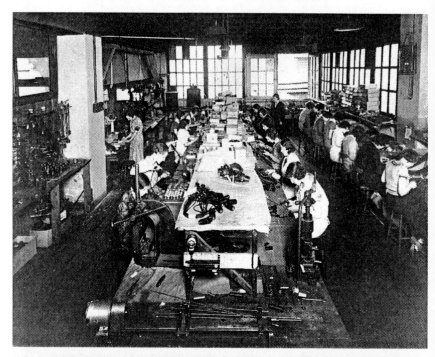

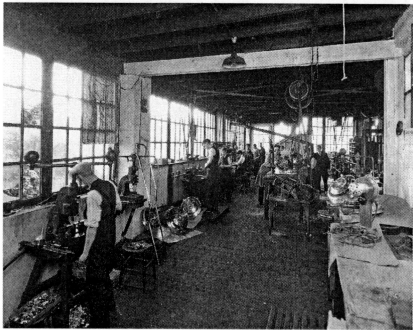

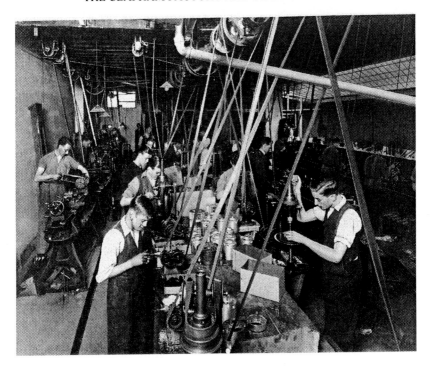

Top (opposite): Room where girls were engaged in wiring and assembling heaters and packaging products such as sachets.

Bottom (opposite): The stamping and pressing room. Some of the 'chandeliers' can be seen on the floor for making the upper part of the permanent waving machines.

Above: Machine shop. Lathes, drills etc. used for making machined parts. Note that at the time, individual motors were not used on the machines, and all were driven by a single very large motor. There may have been an economic reason for this or it may have evolved from early workshops where water was the sole source of power.

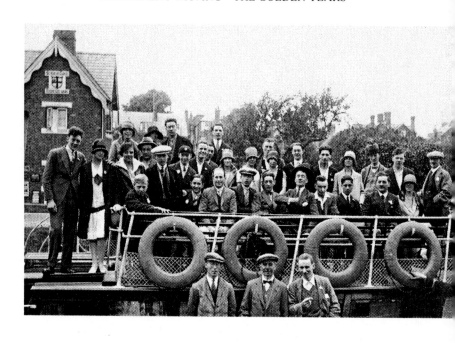

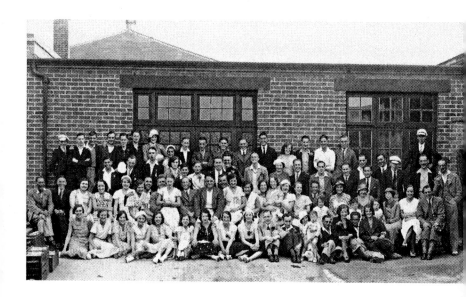

By all accounts, relations with the workers were generally good. However, there were occasional management troubles, specifically one works manager was sacked because he did not get on with the workers. My father seemed to have run the firm with paternal benevolence and the workers must have been grateful to have continued employment at a time when unemployment in Britain and elsewhere in the world was high. An indication of this is that when in 1939 my father proclaimed that he was leaving, many believing that he was starting a business elsewhere in Britain and had asked to go with him.

In keeping with tradition, the company had the usual summer outings and Christmas dinner dances, and some photographs are shown as a social record of the time. These events are a good indication of fashions at the time, - and most of the women have had permanent-waves.

Above, opposite:
Icall outing 28th May 1927, at Sunbury Lock on the Thames. Cloche hats seem to be the fashion.
Front Row: My father (bald) with my brother (17).

Below, opposite:
Icall outing to Margate, 1934. In 7 years, the clothing code has changed markedly. My father (left middle) wearing jacket next to the large gentleman who is the works manager.

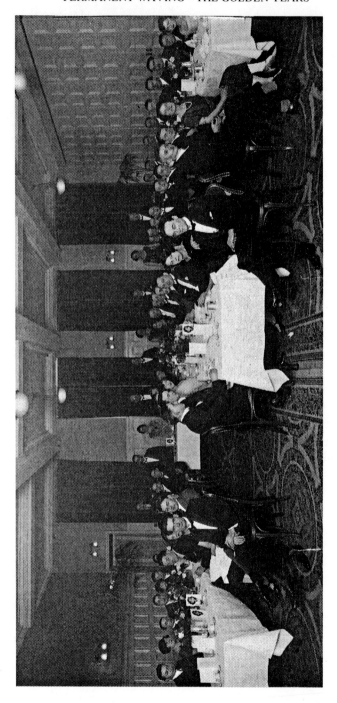

Opposite: The earliest staff Christmas dinner, circa 1923, venue unknown. At the head table, in the middle, are my father and mother and at extreme right with his wife, Mr Bunford, Managing Director of Eugene Ltd who liaised with I. Calvete and was a family friend until the end. Most of the staff from Newman Street and Little St. Andrew Street were men, and women who appear in the picture with them are probably mostly wives or girl-friend. Later, work was outsourced to a place in Camden Town mainly run by women, and these later travelled across London when the firm moved to Clapham, and this indicates a relative satisfaction with their jobs.

While the men carried out the mechanical, heavy work making machines, the girls tended to the winding of heaters and motors, and later the packaging of sachets.

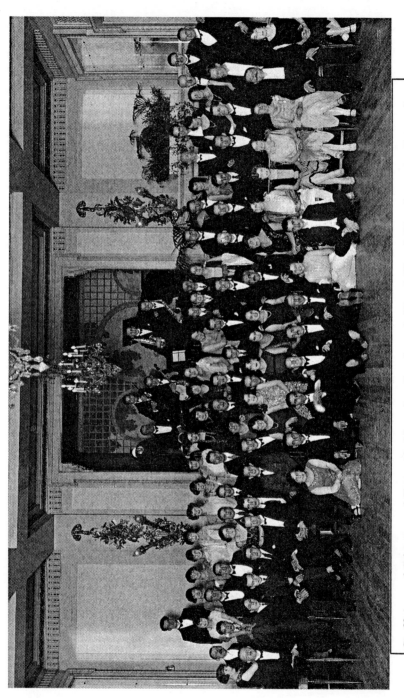

Staff Annual Dinner and Dance held at the Rembrandt Hotel (South Kensington), December, 1926. My father in front, with feet out, next to Mr Martin (moustache).

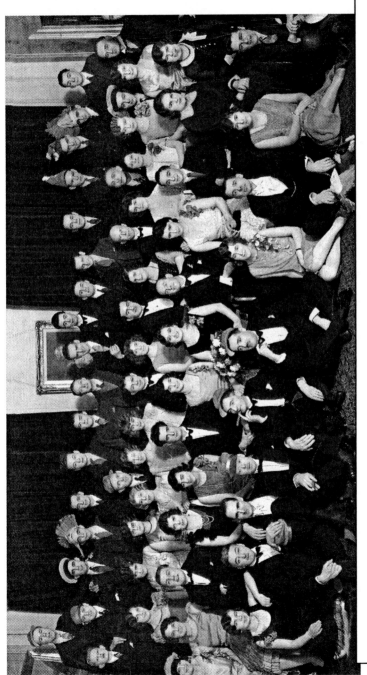

Staff Annual Dinner and Dance held at the Spanish Club, 5 Cavendish Square, December, 1929. My mother, my father, his secretary and my brother are together in the second row. In the front row, fourth from left, Mr Bunford M.D. of Eugene Ltd. and sixth, Martin

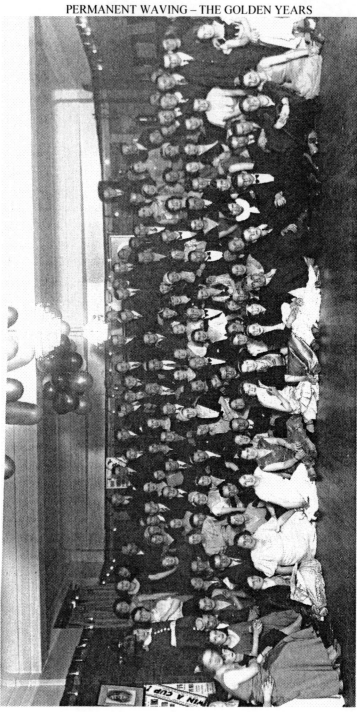

Icall Social, December 1933. This seems to have been a more informal occasion, with few outsiders.

Styles

An innovation, such as permanent waving, can originate from two factors: a physical one which satisfies an existing requirement and a psychological one, which satisfies a desire.

At the turn of the twentieth century, there had been a requirement for some means of waving hair, which until then had been met by Marcel waving. Nessler has the credit for applying an electrical solution to the problem, though I would suggest that it was Calvete that produced a more elegant technical solution to the matter, while it was Eugene who had the initiative to make it such a success. What should be kept in mind is that there was a hidden demand for such a system; for some reason, and for a long time, people preferred wavy hair to straight hair - otherwise, why would wigs always be made with curls? Perhaps it was because people with naturally curly hair were relatively rare, and people with straight hair looked plain.

The psychological factor is one where there is no direct practical need, but for it to materialise the technology must already be in place. Then using this technology to design something new, the latter is offered to the public with the hope that it will create a desire for it. If accepted, it would become the fashion,. By its very nature, fashion is transitory because the desire factor gradually decreases until it becomes mundane. Perhaps there is somewhere a study which relates psychology and fashion, but a search in Google of the two terms together did not come up with any hits

It is not my intention to give a classification of styles during this period, as this can be found in other books, such as Reference 7. Finding examples would not be difficult because by 1930 the vast majority of women would be having some sort of permanent wave. However there would be a range of styles from those by expensive, high-class fashion hairdressers and those produced at hairdressing competitions, to the run-of-the-mill small hairdresser whose aim was to produce an acceptable style with the minimum of complications and expense.

Such was the universality of the permanent-wave, that you have only to look at pictures of women of all social levels, in papers, magazines and films of the 20s and 30s to see examples. Another good place to see them is in present day films and television programmes representing that period to see how the styles have been copied. Agatha Christie programmes are a good example (e.g. Poirot and Miss Marples). And indeed practically every photograph in this book which shows women will confirm that practically all of them had been permanently waved. A few examples of the styles are now included.

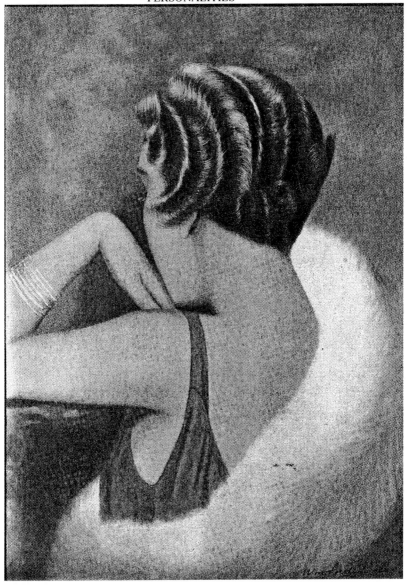

First Prize in a 1932 Competition at the Hairdressing Fashion Fair. Note the deep waves (achieved with a setting lotion and the application of pressure with the fingers to form the waves) and the relatively simple yet elegant style.

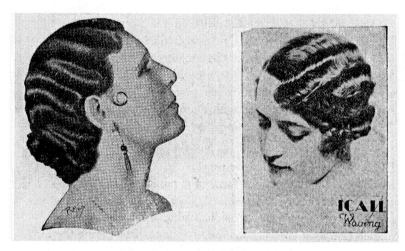

Show Cards were provided free to hairdressers so that they could display them in their windows and provided ideas for styles for their clients. Plates could also be supplied for the hairdresser to print his own cards. "Chosen with extreme discrimination, they are welcomed by your printer. No advertising hairdresser need produce dull literature."

Right, my mother displaying an "Icall" perm on a posh night out.

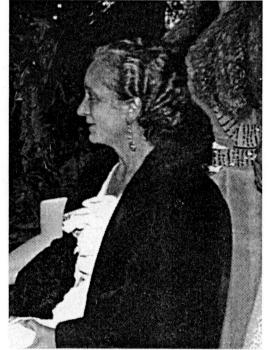

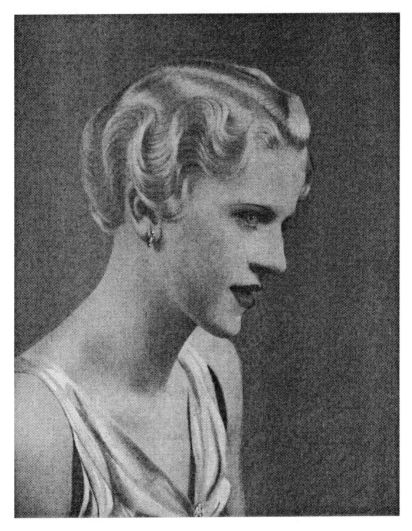

An Evening Coiffure by Eugene (1935)

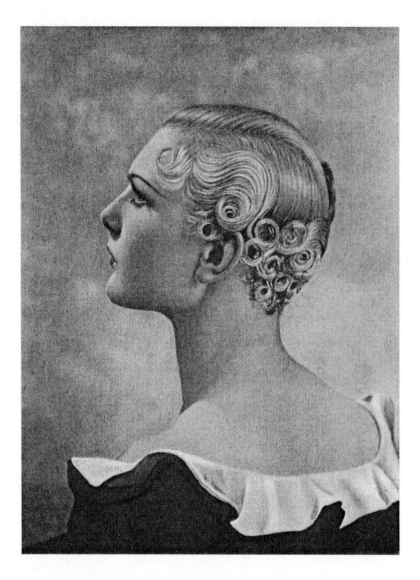

Icall model at an exhibition competition (1935)
demonstrating the so-called plastic style, in which yellow and
mauve pigments were added to the setting lotion, to produce a
spectacular effect.

Personalities

The hairdressing profession has always contained many colourful personalities (and Reference 16 gives a good account of them). This may partly be due to the fact that many, in London at any rate, were foreigners. Also, as Paris was at the time the source of all fashion, it was quite usual for practitioners to imply they had some connection with France, perhaps by adopting French names and certainly by using French terms, such as "salon"

Inevitably, my father formed a wide circle of acquaintances among wholesalers, manufacturers and particularly hairdressers some of which became family friends.

Before the First World War, it was customary for people to work six days a week, only having the Sunday off. After this war, firms, including shops, started allowing their employees to have Saturday afternoons off, a practice known abroad as an "English Saturday". This allowed an extension of leisure activities, and attending football matches on Saturday afternoons became a popular habit. My father, who had made a number of close friends amongst the hairdressing community, and this group attended football matches (mainly Arsenal, but also Tottenham and Chelsea), followed by dinner somewhere (perhaps the Spanish Club) and games of cards.

As I was only a child at the time, I rarely met these people, but this changed due to an exceptional circumstance.

My earliest holidays were when the family went with neighbours to stay in Devon, but in 1926, my father took up British citizenship and in 1927 he obtained a pardon from the Spanish government for his desertion as a conscript. As a result, the family was then free to travel to Spain on an annual holiday and visit relatives. The journey was an arduous one by car, and after a few years, I stopped going because the car journey made me sick. My father used to meet up with one or both his brothers and spent an active week in Pamplona at the San Fermin festival, though none of them was foolhardy enough to run with the bulls. However, this came to a stop in 1936 with the outbreak of the Spanish Civil War, so an alternative had to be found.

It is difficult at this distance in time to establish how it happened, but someone amongst the group of hairdressers who we knew personally had found a farm in Somerset which could accommodate a fair number of residents and it became customary, particularly when there was a Bank Holiday, for a group consisting mainly of fashionable London hairdressers and their families, to travel to Somerset and stay at a farm house in South Cadbury. This happened in the years 1935 to 1939. The names I can still remember are Mr. Laporte (French, Salon at 29 Duke Street, W.1, and Dover Street, Mayfair, which he acquired from Eugene); Mr Georges Veillat (French); Mr. Fern (Fern Barbuto); Mr. Martin (Martí Abella, who was Spanish, 17 Coventry Street), Mr V. Olofson (Notting Hill Gate), Mr Marcel and Mr. Joseph (Wilczewski who was Polish and whose salon was in Sutton) and the inimitable Raymond (who claimed to have been born in Normandy but was probably born in the East End). Mr. Martin was reputed to have invented the 'setting' of permanent waves in the 20s; up till then permed hair was just combed so that it just sat naturally from the perm. Setting the hair, required artistry, placing or pushing the hair in a predetermined way and then setting it under a dryer. This simple technique was universally adopted and led to the elegant styles which would be seen in competitions or amongst the well-to-do. Another hairdresser with whom my father had a strong association was a Spaniard called Tapias whose establishment occupied a whole building in Hanover Square.

146

In retrospect, it is difficult to see why these sophisticated persons with hairdressing salons in the West End of London or the stockbroker belt and accustomed to every comfort would choose this farm, because it was typical of its period. Like most farms at the time (and for that matter, many houses in towns) there was only one toilet and that was at the end of the garden (it was made of wood and had a handle which sprinkled sand when you had finished). There was a tin bath available but I do not think anyone bothered to use it. There was no telephone and a radio which ran off accumulators which were generally flat. There was no electric power so paraffin lamps were used for the main rooms and candles for the bedrooms.

The farm was run by Mr Miller, (very affable, like all his family) who kept a dairy herd which had to be milked twice a day by hand, as there was no electricity for a milking-machine. This had to be done by Mr Miller and his two sons, Harold and Derek, who were about my age, the latter having to fit this activity into their school hours. Mr Miller had no car, but as all visitors came by car, transport was no problem. Mrs Miller, who had three other, younger children as well, had to deal with the domestic arrangements. In particular, this required cooking three times a day for perhaps 25 visitors. This was all done on a paraffin stove, as there was no gas. In spite of the basic nature of the accommodation, it was very comfortable and the food simple but good and plentiful. Meals were taken with great bonhomie and repartee, what you might expect from a group of extrovert, jovial, fashionable hairdressers all sitting at one big table, and work was seldom touched upon. Perhaps it was a relief to escape from the artificiality of the salon and return to the simple life.

Activities, too, were basic. South Cadbury consisted only of a few cottages and the nearest (3 miles) small town was Sparkford. One or two might go to Wincanton for the horse-racing, but golf was generally more popular. The course was fairly isolated and unfrequented so nearly everyone accompanied the players round the course. I used to caddy for my father, and on one occasion, for Martin and Raymond. The men used to go the pub and play skittles, and there was even a dance held in the farm yard. Although my father was the odd man out, being a manufacturer, while all the rest were hairdressers, these were purely social occasions with no attempt at commercial advantage.

Another activity indulged in by the grown-ups was shooting, mainly of rabbits. On one occasion Raymond, I believe, shot a fox, which had to be buried secretly at night as apparently this could have got Mr Miller into trouble as the local hunt did not like this sort of thing. Sometimes, a car would be driven into a field at night and after a spell of waiting, the headlights would be put on and pot-shots taken at the rabbits caught in the lights.

Otherwise the evenings were spent at skittles in the local public house, though of course we children were not allowed in, otherwise everyone gathered together in the light of a paraffin lamp, playing party games and card games, which is how I learned pontoon. Martin and Raymond were great gamblers and sometimes played private card games at which large sums changed hands.

The most colourful individual, and the one who became famous later, was Raymond, born Raymond Bessone, who was the son of a barber and had been a wrestler before taking up ladies' hairdressing. He was about 26 at this time, and had recently opened his own Mayfair salon in 18 Grafton Street, Mayfair with silk ceilings to be followed by other salons at Albemarle Street and elsewhere. He had already developed a reputation for flamboyancy. On one occasion, Raymond created a minor sensation by turning up at the farm with a large, brand new American car, specially imported, complete with American chauffeur. But it was after the war that Raymond became especially notorious and acquired the nickname Mr Teasey-Weasey from his appearances on television, twice won the Grand National and coiffeured many famous ladies, including the Duchess of Windsor and Mrs Attlee. (Reference 12).

Meanwhile, we children, guided by Harold and Derek explored the countryside (there was little else to do). Very nearby, was Cadbury Castle, a large iron age hill fort, said to be the site of Camelot, and which we called Arthur's Castle.

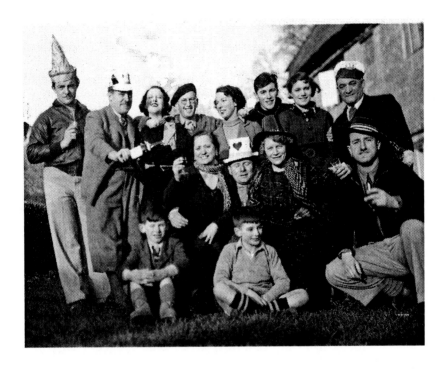

Party outside the farm. Back row from left: Raymond, Martin, Mrs Laporte, my father, unknown, Martin's son and daughter Richard and Carmen, ? Middle row: my mother, ?, Mrs Martin, Laporte. Front: Derek and me.

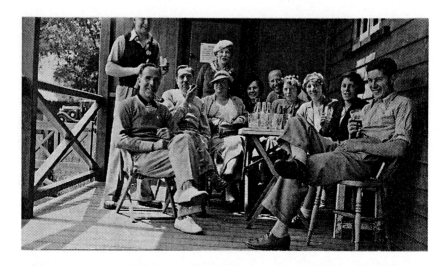

Above: At the Golf Club: Seated from the left: George Veillat, Martin, my mother, Mrs Veillat, Mrs Martin, unknown, the Martins' daughter and son..

Below: The yard of the farm, Mr Miller with his arm round my mother.

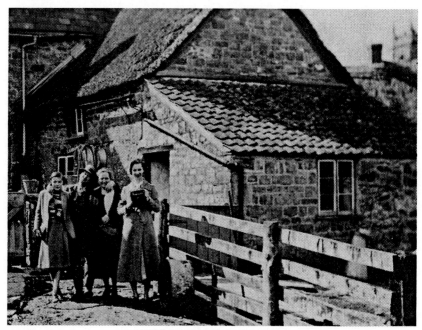

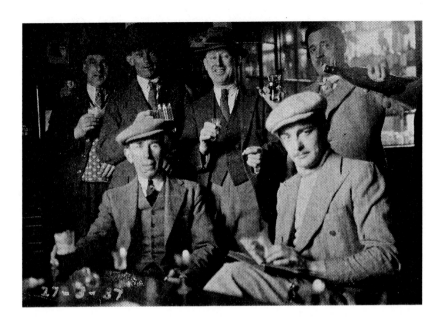

At the local hostelry: Mr Miller in middle, Martin holding bottle over Raymond's head. The latter always tried to appear the elegant sporting gentleman and was very keen on betting. Apart from playing golf (when I once caddied for him), he played cards for money with Martin and frequented the Wincanton races. At some stage he is said to have broken the bank at a Belgian casino and was the only owner to have won the Grand National twice.

Apart from friends, there were also numerous business associates in all branches of the manufacturing and hairdressing professions. A focal point of the latter for the ordinary hairdresser were the wholesalers who supplied everything from machines and dryers to pins, combs and reagents. Two that I was aware of as being important were R. Hovenden and Osborne, Garret & Co (51-54 Frith Street). The latter had the logo Ogee and was the larger organisation, but the founders originally worked for Hovendens.

An annual feature in the hairdressing calendar was the Wholesalers' Dinner. Everyone of importance in the profession who wanted to see and be seen, attended. I remember these occasions as being on a Saturday night, and there was much activity at home as my parents got themselves ready to attend. I discovered that one feature was that a basket was given to every lady attending, which was filled with freebies supplied by the manufacturers: flowers, shampoos, perfumes, cosmetics, brushes, combs and so on, and next morning when I got up and went into my parent's bedroom I would find this basket and examine its fragrant contents. Apparently the presentation of a basket of goodies to celebrities attending a function (e.g. premieres) has now become usual at such events as films premieres and formal events for footballers, pop stars and films stars.

Photograph on opposite page) A Hairdressers' Wholesalers' Dinner about 1930. My parents are sitting at the nearest table to the viewer. My mother is the only woman on the table. On her right is my father and opposite, wearing glasses is Mr. Laporte.

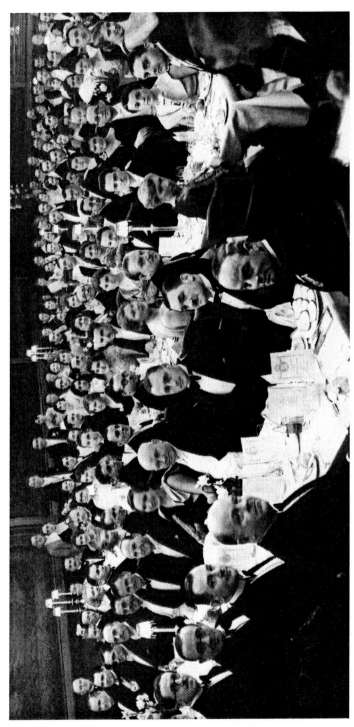

Opposite: The Hairdressers' Wholesaler's Association Dinner was a large and, not surprisingly, a very elegant affair, in which the ladies vied in fashion and hair styles. Here, at the event held at the Mayfair Hotel, Berkeley Street, on Wednesday, 6th February 1935, those attending are apparently waiting to enter the dining hall, holding their drinks. There were some 400 guests, many speeches and a move to unite the Wholesalers' Association with the Hairdressers' Guild, not to mention a band and a cabaret. The luminescent lady on the right is my mother. I, being only 12, spent the night with a family friend. (HJ 1935, p. 652).

Below : A group at the same dinner.   The lady at the back on the left is my mother, and the man next to her with the button-hole is my father. The two to the right are the work's manager and his wife. The man on the right holding a glass is Monsieur Laporte.

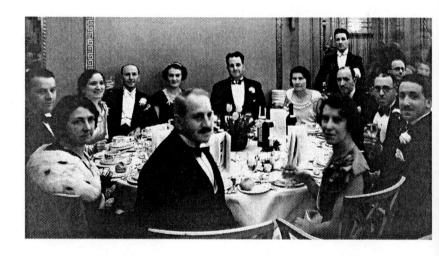

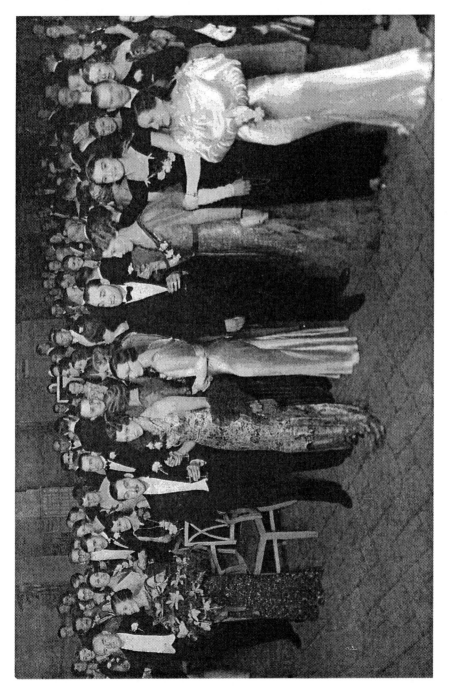

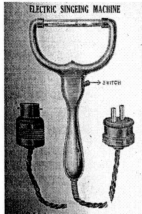
The Electric Singeing Machine.   Note that it was supplied with a two-pin plug or a bayonet fitting. Claiming to be well-insulated, in common with other devices at the time, it was not earthed. The bayonet fitting was used to plug into the light socket, a common practice when houses were ill-provided with electric sockets. (Hairdressers' Weekly Journal, January 1920)

Below: The electric Marcel-waving tongs. An elegant device which should have been a huge success as most hairdressers did Marcel waving, when permanent waving machines were rare, but for some reason it was not followed up.

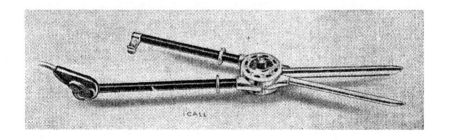

Early Icall Products,
including medical and beauty equipment

As stated earlier, the first product my father invented in this country was an electrical device for sealing letters which had been censored, for use during the First World War. A number of other minor devices followed, such as an electrical cigarette and an electric lighter for gas-stoves, the prototype of which was used satisfactorily at our home during the twenties and thirties. It consisted of a hard carbon rod inset into an ebonite handle, which contained some components, and then connected directly to the mains. To use it, the gas was turned on and the rod briefly rubbed against the burner, the sparks which were formed igniting the gas. It must have saved us a fortune in matches, but apart from the odd unit made for a friend, it was never marketed. Just as well, as by today's standard it might not be considered electrically acceptable, but a similar device is now often installed on gas cookers but which works by means of a piezo-electric system, but ours probably was based on a capacitor in the handle which limited the current on contact with the burner thereby creating sparks..

In January 1920, I. Calvete Ltd started advertising a new product which was simply called an Electric Singeing Machine. It had been the fashion for some time to singe the ends of hair, using a lighted taper, and this service was offered to both sexes. It was believed to have a beneficial effect of thickening the hair and may even have prevented the formation of 'split ends'. The method used was to pass a small lighted taper near to the ends so that they were singed. Different techniques were used, for example, with long hair it might

157

have been twisted into a long roll which was then singed, or with post-war bobbed styles, just combing the ends and applying the flame. Obviously a proper hand-held device gave much greater control over the process and reduced the work and risks of traditional singeing. The product aroused considerable interest, — an order for 250,000 from the USA had to be turned down, perhaps because of other commitments! In any case, the change in styling may have caused the product to be dropped.

In March 1923, my father obtained patent No. 17889 for a device which he registered in May 1924 with the trade-mark Teleswitch. At a time when electric lighting was only beginning to spread as a form of domestic illumination, the Teleswitch was intended to provide several switches in one room to control one electric light. In current practice, the greatest number of switches for the purpose is two, perhaps at opposite ends of a large room, using a two-pole, two-way switch. The advantages claimed for the Teleswitch were a larger number of simple switches could be used and because only a low voltage was used, the system was not only safer, but also unobtrusive because bell wire could be used. In practice, the switches were simple bell buttons, and the light could be switched on or off from anywhere in the room where the bell button had been installed. The controller to which the switches were connected, and shown in the following photograph, could be situated in an un obtrusive place.

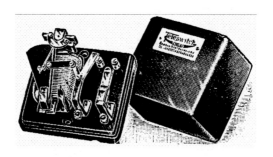

The Teleswitch controller.

An early photograph shows my father demonstrating the bell-push for the Teleswitch, the latter being invisible as it was installed 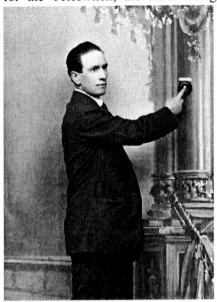 elsewhere where it could not be seen. This photograph seems to have been an early, inexpensive attempt at a publicity photograph taken in an old studio such as those used by the Victorians for family portraits, with a patently false background. Apart from the unlikely case of a bell-push being installed on a column, I understand the bell-push was not connected to anything and was in fact held in position by my father's finger.

There was a considerable interest in the product in professional electrical circles. Unfortunately, like a number of other products, it had to be abandoned because of the demands on hair-dressing equipment. It should be remembered that only recently built houses might have wiring for electricity and suppliers depended on what was available locally. When electricity became more readily available and the difference in tariffs was eliminated, many appliances were run (without earth connection) from the bayonet socket of the light because of the absence of power sockets. Electric irons were popularly used this way as the cord hung out of the way of the ironing action, but radios and fires might be run this way but it was useful to have someone in the house who knew how to repair fuses.

A much more promising idea which was probably not followed up for the same reason, was the electric Marcel-waving tongs. Apart from the poor presentation afforded by the original tongs on top of a gas-burner, it was difficult to judge for how long to heat them to attain the correct temperature. A bit low, and the curl would hardly form, while too hot and they could damage the hair. In addition, the tongs cooled fairly quickly during use and loose their effectiveness.

Both drawbacks were corrected in the electric tongs by maintaining a constant and correct temperature, and also because re-heating was not required, so that the hairdresser could curl the hair at three times the speed of gas-heated tongs. There is no doubt that the expert Marcel waver could achieve excellent results but the advances of permanent waving techniques enabled greater constancy of results and encouraged the development of new styles, but although Marcel waving gradually disappeared, it has reappeared in new forms which enable women to carry out styling at home and the Icall electrical Marcel tongs can perhaps be seen as the forefather of present domestic, electric crimping and styling appliances. Of course, the same principle can be applied to straightening the hair, hence the "hair-straighteners" which are now in use which by simply dragging hair through a heated pad straightens the hair so that it hangs straight down the side of the head. Some of these have ceramic surfaces which give a smooth surface to the surface of the hair as it passes through.

At an early stage, my father became involved in the manufacture of electrical medical equipment which at the time may have looked more promising than hairdressing equipment. The use of electricity in medicine was only just emerging and I. Calvete Ltd developed a considerable range of medical appliances. At a time when medical treatment was mostly palliative, the use of electrical appliances seemed an alternative method of treatment which could be used in the home. In addition. Health and Beauty have always gone hand in hand with Hairdressing, and this was the Age of Modernism in which technical developments and healthy living were supposed to advance hand in hand. Thus, designing, manufacturing and selling

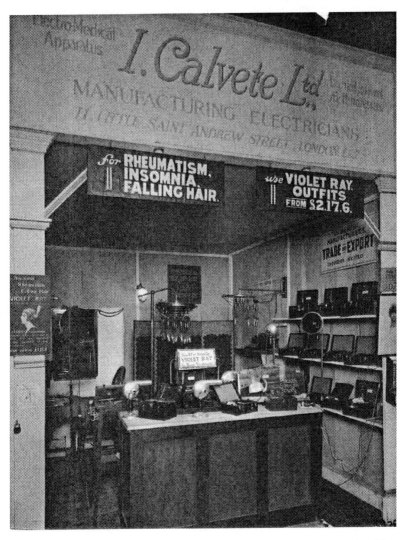

A stand at the Ideal Home exhibition of 1925 in which health or medical equipment was prominent. Note the extravagant claims for the Violet Ray equipment.

However, there are already two permanent waving machines in the background and a hand-held dryer in the front.

this equipment was an important part of Icall business until the early thirties. It can be divided into four classes: ultra-violet light, infra-red light, high frequency treatment and massage.

I. Calvete Ltd made **ultra-violet lamps** which worked on the basis of an arc created by two carbon electrodes. The persons being treated had to wear special goggles to protect the eyes. The treatment was mainly therapeutic as it had been shown that rickets occurred in conditions of poor sunlight. Such conditions would be found mainly in the more northern parts of the country or where the weather was very cloudy, but an important factor was that most industrial cities and towns had a permanent pall of smoke and soot which cut out the sun's ultra-violet rays. An alternative treatment for vitamin D deficiency was the administration of cod liver oil (Vitamin D had not yet been discovered). Rickets has also been reported among dark-skinned immigrants living in a dull climate.

However, sales were only made to hospitals and doctors since legislation had been introduced that ultra-violet equipment was not to be used by 'unqualified' persons. Hairdressers were classed as such, although they could have used it for the treatment of certain scalp complaints such as psoriasis and alopecia. It is interesting to note that before that time, sun-bathing as it was called, for cosmetic purposes was not generally indulged in. From earlier times, ladies "of quality" took every precaution, as a cosmetic procedure, to avoid the sun falling on their skin by wearing long sleeves and hats, and using parasols to preserve their lily-white skin. The reason was that women who acquired a brown face or brown hands were generally exposed to the sun by their work, and were therefore of the lower classes.

It was only in the twenties and thirties that women on the continent created the fashion of being tanned, either because it made them more attractive or implied they had the money to go to the South of France. Today, ultra-violet treatment is mainly used by beauticians to obtain a "tanned" cosmetic effect or, at any rate, to produce some protection before going on an overseas holiday. The light comes from fluorescent tubes without the phosphor coating which in ordinary use would create visible light. The ultra-violet light is more like that of a mercury lamp and because it does not contain some of the shorter-wave lengths, is less dangerous than carbon-arc or solar light and less-expensive to run than the former. But other health aspects have now turned full circle. A reduction in the ozone layer means that higher doses of ultra-violet penetrate the atmosphere and extreme care is now taken to avoid continuous direct sunlight to avoid cancer of the skin. One wonders how much these precautions, such as the use of high-factor sun screens, increase the risk of rickets and, for that matter, affect the later appearance of osteoporosis.

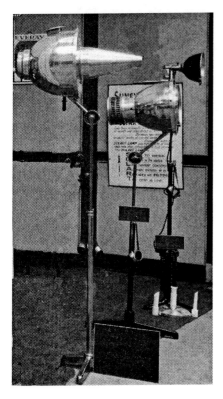

Three of the early models of carbon-arc, ultra-violet ray equipment called Solart.

The two on the left are professional models and the third is for domestic use.

Each has a pair of dark goggles hanging half-way down, to protect the eyes during use.

The Solart No. 2 showing the carbon rods which emitted the ultra-violet light. In the form shown it would be used for general body irradiation or 'tanning'. The accessories enabled the variation of the area covered. The ring could be for treatment of scalp disorders while the 'trumpet' (shown in place above) was for 'cavities', presumably in dentistry.

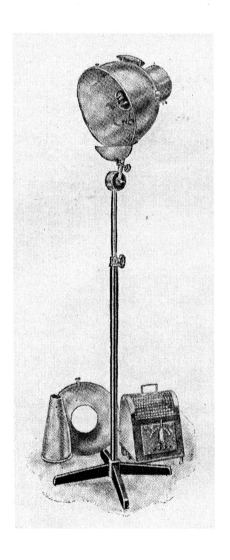

Infra-Red lamps, or "radiant lamps" as they were called, were and are used for the treatment of muscular complaints which is known as diathermy (or 'deep heat'), but does not seem to have any great application in the beauty field. The lamps made by I. Calvete Ltd were similar to those readily available today and were used in the same way.

Right: The professional Radiant Therapy Light, with a 350 W carbon bulb.

Below: An I. Calvete Ltd, portable radiant heat (infra-red) lamp with a 200 W carbon bulb.

Both models could be provided with a red, blue, orange or green filter.

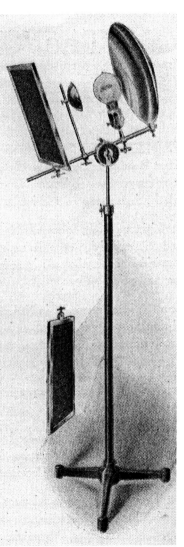

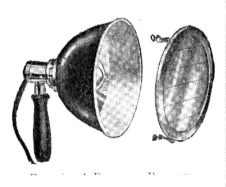

The medical product on which my father placed most emphasis in the early days was the Violet Ray High Frequency machine. The basis of this was a Tesla coil, a self-oscillating coil working at a high frequency and this was discharged through what was called an electrode, but which was in fact a glass envelope containing an inert gas at low pressure, and this was then applied to the part of the body to be treated. To facilitate this, the electrode could be obtained in a variety of shapes according to the part to be treated, but for most purposes a flattened bulb on the end worked well. The gas in the envelope would glow, but only a tingling feeling could be detected and slight redness after 10-15 minutes. The colour of the discharge depended on the gas in the envelope and most frequently was violet, so the phenomenon was called Violet Ray, an unfortunate name as it became confused with ultra-violet light which was totally different. Many extravagant claims were made at the time, but it appears to have been generally harmless, and there is no doubt that in certain cases the stimulated circulation of the blood (hyperaemia) did some good.

My father designed a domestic version called the Everay contained in a wooden box which would hold two or three electrodes and had one or two switches - an on/off/voltage selector and an intensity control. Large numbers of these were made and sold. The high-frequency today would cause havoc with television, radio and telephone systems, but in those days this did not seem to matter. Early displays of the company's products showed large numbers of the Everay with a large assortment of electrodes, including a comb version for treating the scalp.

Occasionally, an example will appear on an antiques programme where it either causes puzzlement or expressions of horror — in fact, it was not alarming in practice and used by many people in their homes. Comprehensive medical books were written showing its use in applications all over the body, and at the time were part of normal medical practice. The devices continued to be displayed and sold at Icall exhibitions into the thirties and this form of treatment may still be in use today in other forms.

166

"Everay" High Frequency
Violet Ray Portable Generator

TYPE B
General
Purposes
Model

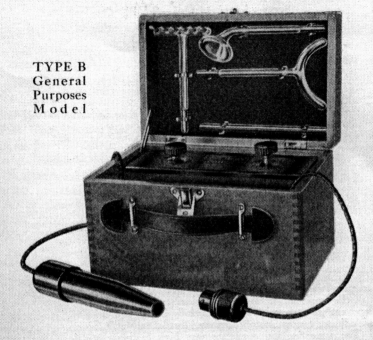

UNIVERSAL VOLTAGE—100 to 250 volts.
For direct and for alternating current.

An "Everay" portable high-frequency (or violet-ray) machine manufactured by I. Calvete Ltd. The lid contained three electrodes, a comb-shaped one for treating the scalp, a straight one for insertion into orifices and the standard bulb which was used for treating surfaces, particularly muscles and joints. The range of voltage and the choice of alternating and direct current is indicative of the variations of supply available in 1926. Only a faint tingle was felt during use, but a slight spark was felt when first applying the electrode. This could be avoided by applying the electrode quickly, but a model was produced with a button in the handle which disconnected the electrode until it was in contact.

Icall also manufactured a number of vibratory devices for massaging muscles in different parts of the body, and the scalp. A general purpose model, the "Meritor", for professional use could be used for massage, manicure and chiropody. Hair clippers could also be supplied as an accessory, and the speed at which it ran could be controlled by a rheostat on the stand.

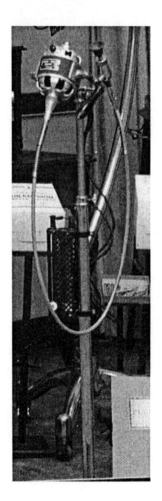

An electric massaging machine more suited to beauty salon and domestic use (the "Vibro") was designed, which originally had an aluminium body, but in 1932 this was replaced by a Bakelite body for even greater lightness. A whole range of applicators could be inserted to give different types of massage.

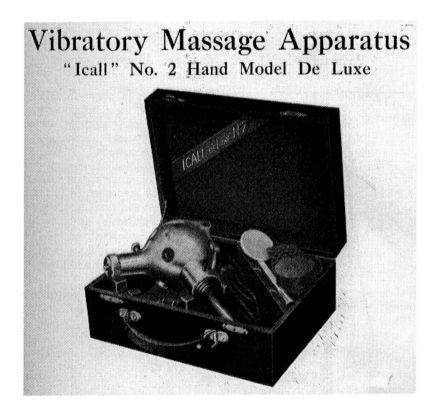

Vibratory Massage Apparatus
"Icall" No. 2 Hand Model De Luxe

A more ambitious massaging machine was for use exclusively on the head. The opinion prevailed that direct massaging of the scalp was beneficial because it stimulated the circulation of blood through the scalp, encouraging the formation of new or healthier hair. This machine was available from 1929 to 1934, but it never proved successful. Perhaps because it was originally given an unhappy choice of name (the "Blud-Rub") but the client would probably be put off by a mechanical device without direct human control.

One of several newspaper reports showed pictures of this device for massaging the head, when it was exhibited in October 1929, at White City. My father at the controls. Most commented on the forbidding appearance of the device. The picture also appeared in papers abroad.

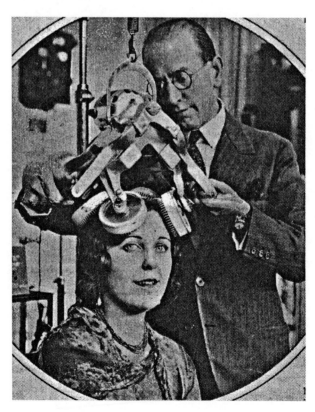

The Second World War - and After

1939. The Spanish Civil War ends and Franco's government is recognised by the British government. Italy seizes Albania. Hitler causes general surprise by signing a pact with the Soviet Union. In September, Germany invades Poland, and Russia occupies East Poland. Britain and France declare war on Germany.

My father resigned from I. Calvete Ltd on the 31st March 1939. The now complete transfer of Icall to Eugene and resignation of my father must have been kept quiet for whatever reason, as I can find no report of this major convulsion at the heart of the business in the Hairdressers' Weekly Journal or anywhere else. I had not long broken up for Easter from the boarding-school I attended and was unaware of what was going on. I had heard of Mr Chamberlain returning from Munich the previous year, with "Peace in our time", but more recently we had been regaled at school with an alarming film called "The Bomber will always get through". Anyway, my education was suddenly cut short and my father had begun to dispose of our house, furniture and car. In May we had our last, short, holiday at the farm in South Cadbury, and in June we set sail in the liner "Reina del Pacifico" to a new life in Ecuador, leaving my brother behind. The liner was nearly empty, but when we made a stop at La Rochelle in France, it was filled to overflowing with German and Austrian Jews. The significance of this was not to dawn on me for quite a long time. When war was declared, we were already living in Quito.

Following the complete take over of I. Calvete Ltd, by the time the war started, production had moved to Eugene, and by 1940 only Greek Street was mentioned in Kelly's Directory as representing Icall. The fate of the factory is not clear but some or all of the equipment was transferred to the Eugene factory.

1940. Germany invades Denmark and Norway, and later France which soon capitulates. British and French troops evacuated from Dunkirk. Germany starts bombing raids across the country and in September causes huge damage during the "Blitz". Following the Battle of Britain, German bombers then concentrated on other cities in the country.

1941. Clothes and food rationing. U.S.A. enters the war.

1942. Battles of Stalingradin, Russia and El Alamein, North Africa/

1944 D-Day (6 June) landings in Europe. The preparations for the largest land invasion ever undertaken on the beaches of Normandy were huge. Of special interest are the two Mulberry harbours (each the size of Dover) which were built to facilitate the landing of large amounts of heavy material and troops. The scale of the project was enormous and was in danger of over-stretching the capacity of the UK's civil engineering industry. From late summer of 1943 onwards three hundred firms were recruited from around the country employing 40,000 to 45,000 personnel at the peak. Their task was to construct 212 caissons ranging from 1672 tons to 6044 tons, 23 pier-heads and 10 miles of floating roadway in a period of about 9 months. Because man-power was very short, men from trades and backgrounds not associated with the construction industry were drafted in and given crash courses appropriate to their work. Many were from the service industries, such as waiters and hairdressers.

1944 also saw the start of attacks by V1(flying bombs or doodle-bugs) of which 2,340 hit London, causing 5,475 deaths, and 16,000 injured. These were followed by V2 supersonic rockets.

1945 End of World War II.

In April 1946, we returned to Britain to find a country devastated by war. Some three million homes had been damaged or destroyed and industry was trying painfully to convert back to peace-time production. Shortages were if anything greater than during the war, and there was bread rationing, something which had not been necessary even during hostilities. Luxuries like hairdressing continued to be low priority. Apart from the absence of hostilities, conditions during the period between 1939 and 1950 were hardly better than during the war, and is difficult to describe in hairdressing terms. The feeling I get is that most women managed the best they could with their hair, excepting perhaps older and better off women in the cities who continued to have their hair attended to. One can imagine that during the war, little by little, hairdressing equipment would break down and replacements would be unobtainable. During the war, practically the only major manufacturer still advertising in the HJ was Macdonald.

Some waving machines were made after the war, but the big names had gone and hairdressers were using rollers heated separately and then applied, a variant of the old "falling heat" method. Eugene Ltd. and I. Calvete Ltd continued to exist as companies but they were practically only shell companies. Eugene consulted my brother on cold-waving and in 1955 they were advertising demonstrations of this system but only hairdryers in the way of equipment. The advent of cold waving had added a new and versatile tool to the hairdresser's armoury. The war had virtually done for the old systems and there was no coming back, and the swinging sixties brought in a new generation of hairdressers.

Of course, my father never returned to the manufacture of hairdressing equipment, but he did acquire a hairdresser's and tobacconists in Sunbury-on-Thames, which he ran for a few years until he retired to Spain. He died in 1965 in Valencia.

My brother James left the firm shortly after the start of war and he had practical engineering skills which were put to use in war work.

After the war, he worked for a short time (1947-48) with Hovendens in Berners Street, a link which had existed since the earliest days. One of the first products he had to sell were the first kits of cold-waving systems for sale at £10 each, to professional hairdressers, a sure sign that things were changing. Then he spent the years 1948 to 1955 managing the hairdressing salons and gift-shops of the Imperial Group of hotels in Russell Square.

I joined Imperial Chemical Industries and stayed there until I retired. It never occurred to me that perhaps I would write up the hairdressing events of my childhood. One of the interesting aspects of this task has been visiting the places where these events took place.

The first was the workshop at 46 Newman Street. It still stands and now houses a Tanning and Beauty Salon. I wonder if those within realise that early ultra-violet equipment was manufactured there. Perhaps there should be a blue plaque on the wall, stating that this was where electric permanent waving really was born! Then there is 11 Little St. Andrew Street WC2, in which serious production first started. The name of the street no longer exists, and at some stage it was re-named Monmouth Street. The ground floor has been joined to the ground floor of the next building on the corner to form a modern coffee-shop. The Ivy Restaurant is still around the corner.

The showroom at 52 Dean Street, still exists and the ground floor is today occupied by the Bank of East Asia Ltd. overlooking Shaftesbury Avenue. The last showroom at 15 Greek Street and which saw the final disappearance of the company, is still there and is now occupied by a Thai Restaurant. Nearby at No. 25 the famous French patisserie Maison Bertaux is still there.

The Clapham factory no longer exists. If in London one sees a row of old houses which is continuous except for a number of newer ones placed in the middle, it is a good indication that some of the houses were destroyed in the blitz. It looks as if this has happened in North Street, Clapham, and there is a strong probability that the factory was destroyed during the "blitz", but I have been unable to find any record of the event. As so much was going on at the time it was unlikely to be reported - in any case, such information would not be made public as it might help the enemy. The "blitz" did huge damage to London, mainly in the City and East End where the docks were, but strategic targets elsewhere were also attacked. The factory was only a mile from Clapham Junction, the largest railway junction in the world and vital for the war effort, and so was heavily attacked by the Germans, with numerous fatalities, and so was very likely destroyed in 1940, though one cannot exclude the possibility of destruction by a V1 or V2 in 1944. The area was one in which the government built large air-raid shelters for the population because of its vulnerability.

On the other hand, the Eugene factory survived the war but its business did not. As a registered business, Eugene continued to exist as indeed did I.Calvete Ltd, but not with any notable commercial activity, and it is apparent that the old technology was stone dead, and attempts to breath life back into it were pointless. The company boards met annually, but were short of ideas. My brother was invited to the Eugene factory and questioned about cold-waving and the company had also shown interest in a method in which heating was accomplished by chemical means (a method which went back to the early days, but had never taken off). Similarly, on the 1st July 1954, the Hairdressers' Journal (the term Weekly had by now been omitted) contained an advertisement headed "Icall COLDWAVE"., and went on "Lotion 2/6 per bottle, Neutraliser 6d per tablet.......Obtainable from all Wholesalers or direct from: I. Calvete Ltd., 90 Avenue Road, Acton, London W.3." Evidently someone thought it was still possible to extract some prestige from a company which I had thought had ceased to trade 15 years before.

The fact of the matter was that a new clientele served by a new race of hairdressers found that they could work with the simplest of equipment, most of which would be produced in a modern, compact design which could almost equally be used in the home and the salon. The only large piece of equipment which is almost exclusive to the salon is the hood-dryer, and this is not seen in the numbers that they were.

Karl Nessler died the 22nd January 1951 in the United States (See Appendix VIII).

During the whole of this study I have emphasised how the name of Eugene dominated the whole of the hairdressing market during this period.   It is a pity that there appears to be no other biographical study of the gentleman or his activities on which one can draw.   I have attempted to cover every aspect which was available because of his association, and later competition, with my father. Nevertheless, much information is elusive and so much of the following which concerns him is fragmentary and in some cases speculative.   My feeling was that he was not a well man and he took the opportunity in 1936 to make Eugene a public company, and shares were eagerly purchased by the public, particularly hairdressers, because they seemed such a gilt-edged security.   This cashing-in of his assets would have made him a rich man and enabled him to take things easy.   I have been told that he died in a Canadian hotel in 1955.   Perhaps he went to Canada to get away from the war.   But the story takes another twist.   He had a son, who while a student at Yale University, inherited his father's estate of $400,000.   When Eugene Jr. refused the inheritance, the trustees of the estate insisted he take it, and even took him to court to force him to accept the money.   In an unprecedented case held in New York City, Judge William T. Collins reluctantly ruled that the young man had a legal right to reject the $400,000. The order legally cut off the 22-year-old student from all future interest in the family fortune, leaving him without income.

Many of the famous hairdressers of the period retired about now, but there was one great survivor and that was Raymond.   His appearances on television made him widely known and it is said that by 1955, his shampoo sachets were selling at a rate of a million a week, enabling "all those women who can't come to me to get at least a little bit of me." (Ref. 12).   I note that in April 1976 he was advertising for a manager for his Windsor salon under the name

Teasy-Weasy (rather than Raymond) a name he acquired from a mannerism on television. He died in 1992 at the age of 80, so when I knew him in 1936 he was just 24 and on the brink of his career.

In the thirties, no ladies' hairdressing salon would be without it "chandelier"-type permanent-waving machine or machines, with hairdressers proficient in their use, and the names Icall and Eugene would have been prominent everywhere. Now these machines are the dinosaurs of the hairdressing profession and very unlikely to return., so much so that they are totally unfamiliar to the public. Doubtless there will still be one or two gathering dust at the back of some store or garage, but the only one I have been able to trace is that at the Museum of London.

If seen today, their very appearance causes puzzlement, amusement and even horror. I hope I have shown that they were quite simple machines used successfully and safely by most ladies' hairdressers on a great proportion of the female population, to create simple but elegant styles which were typical of the era and used at every level of society.

As I see it, the external appearance of a woman depends on clothes, make-up and hair. Of these, only clothes has any permanence. Thus repeated visits to the hairdresser are generally necessary if any elaborate attempt at style is desired, unless a very simple one (such as straight hair) is adopted. Thus there is a direct link between the creator and the client which generally does not exist with clothing. In addition, the short-lived nature of hair styles means that they only survive in pictures so while there are innumerable displays of real clothing in museums, there is no equivalent for hair-styles. This may account for a shortage of displays of old hairdressing equipment.

Today, there is a very great selection of electric appliances, mostly inexpensive and relatively small, for use in the home or in the salon. *Straighteners* have no equivalent in pre-war days that I know of and there is a great variety of these including models with ceramic and other surfaces to give greater gloss or less resistance when pulling hair through; some may be used on wet hair. (I have it on good authority, that before the appearance of straighteners, a home method used, particularly by members of certain ethnic groups, was to iron the hair by using a domestic electric iron, which would work on the same principle but would not be anywhere near as convenient.)

Wavers and *stylers* heat the hair in a range of configurations, including so-called brushes, rollers and helical curlers. These are the modern, electrical equivalents of the old Marcel wave.

Rollers, which can be heated, or applied to moist hair which is then dried. These seem to be descendants of the classic rollers shown in old films where women (generally working class) wear them during the day, perhaps covered with a head-scarf.

Hand-held Dryers, with styling accessories. These are a world removed from the pre-war variety which were just used for drying, and because they are lighter and smaller lend themselves as a tool for styling the hair. While at one time salons would have a row of helmet-type dryers to cope with the large number of women having their hair dried, now there will be one or none, replaced by a rack of hand-dryers.

It is said that fashion runs in cycles and so one can ask whether the old styles fancied by all levels of society in the pre-war days will return. Certainly in the 70s and 80s, footballers and film stars rushed to have their hair permed, but these styles had little in common with the pre-war ones. Rather than permanent waving they were more like permanent curling of the whole head so that the final effect was one of a large sphere of random curly hair with no general pattern. Seen today, this exaggerated style seems comical and I cannot see that returning in a hurry. On the other hand, the original permanent waving combined simplicity and elegance. There seems to be ample scope for variations within the limitations it imposed. Styles based on them could readily be created, but using modern methods of waving. If people became familiar with them, I think they could readily adapt to the modern world. Present styles seem to be set for ever, but the fickleness of fashion is notorious. Perhaps there is some daring stylist out there who could promote them on a fashion cat-walk or open a Retro hairdressing salon. I am not sure we have seen the end of them.

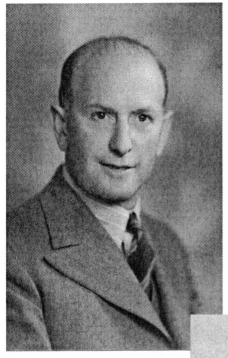

My father, Isidoro Calvete, about 1930, when he was Managing Director of the Company when it was at about its peak. He was short-sighted, but avoided wearing his glasses whenever possible, and kept them in his breast pocket. He was a Fellow of the Institute of Electrical Engineers, a founder member of the Spanish Club and a devoted member of Rotary International for as long as he was able to participate.

My brother James, (about the same time as above), started work at I.Calvete Ltd in Little St. Andrew Street, where he became familiar with the products and their method of manufacture He also acquired some skill in ladies' hairdressing and so became ideally suited as a salesman, covering the important London area (until war broke out) which included, of course, the West End, where he met and knew many of the prestigious hairdressers of the day.

179

... and finally, an advertisement from the January 1935 edition of the HJ, which is the one that in my opinion best encapsulates the peak reached by the techniques and technology of the period:

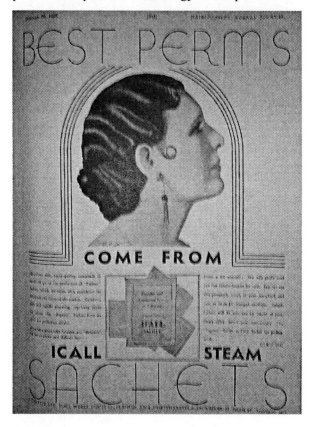

(1) The graphics are all in Art Deco, a style which affected all fields of the arts and design, but which died down after 1939. Occasionally it has reappeared and reappears in certain fields, - and numerous fonts, such as those shown, can be downloaded from the internet.

(2) The importance of sachets as a means of speeding up the perming process and reducing labour is evident, and the presence of water prevented overheating and produced soft waves safely.

(3) A typically simple but elegant hair style of the time, complete with kiss curl, the product of twenty years of development.

References and acknowledgements

1.   I. Calvete   Personal diaries, 1921 - 1939

2.   J. Bari-Woollss.   The Manual of the Permanent Waver. Westminster City Publishing Co. August, 1934.

3.   Robert Pols. Dating old photographs, FFHS, 2nd edition 1995.

4.   Histelec News, December 2003 on Sebastian de Ferranti and the Deptford Power Station .
http://www.swehs.co.uk/docs/news25su.html

5.   Nessler Self-published, 1926. This book was authored by the original inventor of permanent waving for hair (1905), Charles Nessler of C. Nestle Company. Illustrated with   drawings,
diagrams, and vintage black-and-white photographs. All about hair types and how to curl hair using the circuline process.

6.   The Hairdressers' (Weekly) Journal, originally for "Hairdressers, Wigmakers and Perfumers".   This periodical was issued weekly from 1881, published by Osborne and Garret, the wholesalers, and became monthly in January 1949 as the Hairdressers' Journal and Hairdressers Journal International in May 1976, with a modern presentation and colour illustrations, published by Reed Information Ltd, Sutton. It was the main publication for the profession until the present day. At 125 years, this must be

amongst our longest running publications While before the war, exhibitions were run by various newspapers such as the Daily Mail and the Daily Sketch, and organisations, such as the British Industries Federation, Hairdressing Awards and Exhibitions are now organised by the Journal. Copies of the Journal from January 1905 can be seen at the library of the London College of Fashion.

7.   Ed. Gilbert A. Foan / J. Bari-Woolls   The Art and Craft of Hairdressing. Pitman, 1938. An essential reference for anyone researching the development of both men's and ladies' hairdressing up to the date of publication. Odd copies are available in the second-hand market but they may be expensive. There are various editions and confusion can be caused by the fact that the publishing dates are not shown and that there are two publishers. I found that the British Library holds 10 copies of the book, in four editions, printed in Britain by, Sir Isaac Pitman, and a U.S. company, New Era. Dates of publication are presumably the years in which the Library received the book, although the Bari-Woolls version was being advertised for sale in the HJ in January 1939:

1st Ed	1931	Foan	Pitman	661 pp
1st Ed	1933	Foan +	New Era	629 pp
2nd Ed	1936	Foan + Bari Woollss	Pitman	624 pp
2nd Ed	1936	Foan + Bari Woollss	New Era	623 pp
3rd Ed	1950	Foan + Wolters	Pitman	663 pp
4th Ed	1958	Foan + Wolters	New Era	530 pp
4th Ed	1963	Foan + Wolters	Reprint	

The gap between 1936 and 1950 is probably due to the war. Foan died on Thursday 19th February 1931, before the second edition, hence the change of editor. His death was extensively reported in the HJ to which he had also been a continuous technical contributor. He also played an important part in hairdressing professional organisations.

The three editors give a cross-section of the history of permanent waving. By the time the first edition came out in 1931, permanent-waving was barely covered. The second edition in 1936 gave considerable coverage and the names Eugene and Calvete were generously represented. When the final editions came out, these references had virtually vanished.

8.   J. Bari-Woollss. The Manual of the Permanent Waver. Westminster City Publishing Co. August, 1934.

9.   "4. Infrared and Raman Studies of Skin and Hair: A review of cosmetic spectroscopy by K Martin, The Internet Journal of Vibrational Spectroscopy Vol 3 Ed 2 2004, 45 references.

10.   British Patent Specification 422,439, 11th January 1935. "Improvements in Electric Heaters for Waving and Curling the Hair". I.B.Calvete. [Gives a detailed description and drawing of the latest improved heater].

12.   Daily Telegraph Book of Obituaries. A celebration of eccentric lives. 1995.

13.   Deptford Power Stations - South Western Electricity Historical Society (Histelec News No. 25)

14.   Appeal District Court of the United States by Eugene Limited against the Nestle-Le Mur Company. Infringement of Eugene Patent 1,266,879. Two attached coaxial heaters.

15   "What is the relative value in UK pounds?" L H Officer quoted in EH.NET (c) 2004.C.

16.   Caroline Cox   Good Hair Days - A History of British Styling. Quartet Books, 1999. An excellent and readable book giving the history and personalities of hairdressing.

17.   "Current research on ethnic hair" by A Franbourg, P Hallegot, F Baltenneck, C Toutain and F Leroy. Journal of the American Academy of Dermatology, June 2003, pp 8115-8119. 16 references. (Available on internet).

18. 1920s London, Museum of London Exhibition November 2003 to July 2004, Exhibition Guide.

19. Modernism 1914-1939. Victoria and Albert Museum Exhibition, April to July 2006 , Exhibition Guide.

20. Electro-Medical Apparatus and Icall Electrical Specialities. (Catalogue, 1926, 36 pages).
Medical Electricitry (Catalogue1937, 16 pages)

21. I. Calvete Ltd. Permanent Waving Equipment, 1934 (Catalogue, 1934, 32 pages).

22 Eugene F. Suter, The Eugene Method. Technical Instructions Personally Supervised By Eugene F. Suter, Eugene Ltd.. 1928. First Edition. Flexible black cloth with attractive silver printed cover. Discusses the technique of "permanent waving" developed by the author. Illustrated with drawing and photos. 93 pages

23 Basque children webpage
www.spanishrefugees-basquechildren.org

24 "The Eylure Story - Tiddlywinks 'n' undies" by Geraldine Aylott (An account of the emergence of a world-wide business in artificial eyelashes in Welwyn Garden City, Herts, England).

My acknowledgements are gratefully given to:

My brother James, the only professional link I have been able to find with direct knowledge of permanent-waving events of the period and whose experience on the subject has been invaluable and unique.

My daughter Claire who instigated the book and has made valuable suggestions.

The help and encouragement of Katherine Baird, Librarian, London College of Fashion, source of the Hairdressers' Weekly Journal (http://vads.ahds.ac.uk/ixbin/).

The kind permission of the Editor of Hairdressers' Journal International to reproduce items from early numbers of that Journal.

Appendix 1

Subtleties of the hair-winding process.

As described in Reference 8, the geometry of hair-waving is not as obvious as it may seem. In naturally curly hair, the hair is formed and grows out of the follicle at a different rate round the follicle, so that it emerges rather like a cork-screw, a helix which is three-dimensional.

In the case of Marcel waving, if the method described in Reference 5 is used, a length of hair held by a comb is pressed between the comb and the scalp with a pair of Marcel tongs and then moved parallel to the comb or the line of the hair, the tendency will be to form a two-dimensional wave, which can lay flat on the head.

Permanent waving, by winding helically on to a curler, produces a geometry which is rather more like naturally wavy or curly hair. (However the use of the word 'permanent' can be questioned because as the hair grows and is cut, the wave gradually disappears.)

An important factor in permanent-waving is what is called the overlap. When winding a lock of hair, subsequent turns can lie at a varying distance from the previous one. If this distance is zero, the hair is wound on itself and the hair will end up as a tight curl - this happens when using a croquignole system. If the overlap is only partial, the hair being wound travels along the length of the curler. For best, results, it was customary to have a 50% overlap of the hair, which produced the required wave.

Some believed that when winding on to a curler, the hair should be in tension for the best results, and curlers were sometimes designed so that the hair could be tensed after winding. However, in the opinion of Bari-Woollss, the tension plays little part, the curling being effected by the heat and the steam. This is just as well because in a lock with many hairs, all of different length, it would be impossible to ensure uniform tension.

By winding on a curler, the hair is produced as a helix or coil, but the waving effect was achieved by flattening this coil. If the coil is slightly stretched, the peaks of the coil flatten equally on either side produced a true wave going evenly up and down. On the other hand, if the coil was pushed sideways, each turn of the coil would rest on the following one, producing a totally different effect, achieved by setting the hair.

The illustration on the front cover of this book gives examples of the various possible forms: The upper head shows waved hair; the bottom left shows curls; the bottom right shows a flat curl as produced by a croquignole curler; while next to the face there are two "kiss-curls".

Appendix II

The following extract is taken from "The Times" of the 16th March 2006.

The perm still making waves 100 years on

BY SIMON DE BRUXELLES

IT IS quite possibly the only thing that the singer Madonna and the Argentinian footballer Diego Maradona ever had in common: the perm.

Now, when it seemed that the world had waved goodbye to the preferred hairstyle of Seventies footballers and Brian May, the perm is making a comeback in the year of its 100th anniversary.

Since the start of the millennium women have been asking their salons to straighten their hair for a "Rachel". Now Madonna sports a brand-new perm and the diminutive Seventies pop singer Leo Sayer and his mass of curls have been resurrected.

Fortunately women asking their stylists for a "Sienna Miller" or a Madonna-style flick are unlikely to have to endure the tortures inflicted in the name of beauty when the permanent wave was invented by an émigré German hairdresser in 1906.

Karl Nessler gave the first public demonstration of his perm machine at his salon in Oxford Street, London. He had experimented on his wife, Katharina, whose devotion was such that he was able inadvertently to burn off all her hair and scald her scalp not once, but twice.

The guinea pig had her hair wrapped tightly around 12in-long, heated brass rods connected to an electric chandelier. A system of weights and pulleys kept the 2lb bars from coming into contact with her scalp. The hair was saturated with sodium hydroxide and the rods heated to 100C for five hours. At the end of her ordeal Katharina possessed a head of brand-new curls.

Nessler, who had moved to London in 1901, was interned as an enemy alien on the outbreak of the First World War. In 1915 he escaped to New York, taking his invention with him. He discovered that copies of the device were already in use but few worked properly. He set up shop and soon owned a chain of salons in New York, Chicago, Detroit and Philadelphia.

It was not until 1938 that the first "cold wave" chemical perm, requiring neither heat nor a machine, was invented. It was a vast improvement on the electric perm, which caused the hair to become dry and brittle.* Nessler died in 1951, more than 20 years before the fashion he had started took the world by storm.

On the football pitch Kevin Keegan epitomised the style adopted by 1970s footballers. Since then, though they may not wish to be reminded of it, stars such as David Bowie, Catherine Zeta-Jones, Meg Ryan, Martin Shaw and Jon Bon Jovi have worn perms.

In the 1980s the "bubble perm", a head of tight curls, was all the rage and was adopted by the group Bananarama and Kylie Minogue. The end of the century appeared to herald the demise of the perm as women opted for a more natural look or tried to emulate style made famous by the actress Jennifer Aniston as Rachel in *Friends*.

Jo O'Neil, the international technical education director for the Toni & Guy chain of salons, predicts a renaissance for the perm. "It has been in and out of fashion over the years, and has taken a lot of criticism, but it's a legendary look," he said. "It was originally developed to give support and hold to a blow dry — the curly effect was just a side-effect, but this developed into an iconic style statement.

"Over the years it has relaxed and is now all about creating movement and texture. New technology allows you to put movement into the hair that will fade away rather than being cut away. The perm has, at last, come of age."

*Author's Notes: I do not believe it has been shown that traditional waving is worse for hair than cold-waving. If properly carried out so that the hair does not dry out, the temperature is automatically controlled at 100°C. The chemicals used were relatively mild compared to those in cold-waving, and there is no reason to suppose that the hair will become dry and brittle. Note that although Nessler is mentioned, Eugene is not mentioned, although he was much more influential in the cause of permanent waving.

Appendix III
Wikipedia Entry on Permanent Waving

This extract quoted verbatim and without comment, gives the story from a U.S. angle and does not even mention the events in London after Nessler left. At a time when travel between the continents of America and Europe and other forms of communication were slow, development to some extent occurred independently. Exploitation of foreign markets was not so easy either. I. Calvete made forays into Europe, particularly Germany and France, and made an attempt at Argentina, but people in many countries copied existing models rather than importing them. Eugene with a branch in New York did seem to have tried attacking the U.S. market, and defending his patent of 1918 (See Appendix IV).

The last reference, getting a perm in 1950, is particularly illuminating.

Taken from *"http://en.wikipedia.org/wiki/Permanent_wave"*

History

The first chemical treatment for curling hair that was suitable for use on people was invented in the year 1905 by the German hairdresser Karl Nessler (1872-1951). The first public demonstration took place on October 8, 1906, but Nessler had been working on the idea since 1896. Previously, wigs had been set with caustic chemicals to form curls, but these recipes were too harsh to use on human skin. His method, called the spiral heat method, was only useful for long hair. The hair was wrapped in a spiral around rods connected to a machine with an electric heating device. Sodium hydroxide, a strong alkali, was applied and the hair was heated (212°F; 100°C or more) for an extended period of time. The process used about twelve, two-pound brass rollers and took six hours to complete. These hot rollers were kept from touching the scalp by a complex system of countering weights which were suspended from an overhead chandelier and mounted on a stand. His first experiments were conducted on his wife, Katharina Laible. The first two attempts resulted in completely burning her hair off and some scalp burns, but the method was perfected and his electric permanent wave machine was patented in London in 1909. It subsequently went into widespread use.

Nessler had moved to London in 1901, and during World War I, the British jailed Nessler because he was German and forced him to surrender his assets. He escaped to New York City in 1915, buying passage on a steamship under an assumed name. In New York, he found that hundreds of copies of his machine were in use, but most did not work well and were unreliable. Nessler opened a shop on East 49th St., and soon had salons in Chicago, Detroit, Palm Beach, Florida and Philadelphia. Nessler also developed a machine for home use that was sold for fifteen dollars.

After World War I, short hair came into vogue. Because Nessler's method wrapped the hair in a **spiral** along the rods, it couldn't be used with short hair and alternate systems began to be developed. The **croquignole** method, where the hair is wrapped straight up the rod from the ends to the scalp, was invented in 1924 by a Czech hairdresser, Josef Mayer. It quickly became popular because it could be used with many different lengths of hair. Also during this time, a machine-less method that applied preheated clamps over the wrapped rods was invented, but it still used the strong alkali solution.

In 1931, at the Midwest Beauty Show in Chicago, Ralph I. Evans and Everett G. McDonough showed a heatless system for the first time. Their method used bi-sulphide solution and was often applied at the salon, left on while the client went home and removed the next day, leading it to be called the **overnight wave**.

While the later methods were improvements on the original, all of those mentioned above used very strong alkali solution, tight wrapping, long developing times and more often than not caused hair damage and scalp burns.

Modern perms

In 1938, Arnold F. Willatt invented the cold wave, the precursor to the modern perm. It used no machines and no heat. The hair was wrapped on rods and a reduction lotion was applied ammonium thioglycolate. This chemical breaks open the disulfide linkages between the polypeptide bonds in the keratin (the protein structure) in the hair. The disulfide bonds give hair its elasticity, and can be reformed with chemicals. Next, an acid neutralizer lotion was applied, (hydrogen peroxide), to close the disulfide bridges again and the hair was reformed to the shape of the rod. The entire process took 6-8 hours at room temperature.

Perms today use this method with sodium thioglycolate instead of ammonium thioglycolate, at a pH of 8 to 9.5. This method takes only 15-30 minutes until the neutralizer is applied to bring down the pH and rebond the hair. [I believe the rebonding is effected by an oxidising agent, eg peroxide, rather than with an alkali. - L.G.C.]

In the 1970's, **acid perms** were invented. These use glycerol monothioglycolate instead and contain no ammonia. They are sometimes called **buffered waves**. This perm is slower but gentler to the hair. Heat is usually added by placing the client under a dryer, after covering the wrapped head with a plastic cap. The reaction is endothermic and the additional heat causes the pH to rise to 6.9 to 7.2.

Other types of modern perms include exothermic perms, which are self timing and self heating; and neutral, or low pH, thioglycolate free perms.

The **reverse perm** straightens the hair instead of curling it. The same chemical methods can be used for this, but the hair is not wrapped around rods. This process is commonly used by African-Americans and others with naturally curly hair.

Technical considerations

There are two parts to a perm, the physical action of wrapping the hair, and the chemical phase. Both of these can affect the result. Important variable in the physical part are what type of rod is used, how the hair is wrapped and how end papers are used. The two most common types of rods are straight and concave; each giving a different curl effect. The wrapping method is either spiral or croquinole, and various types and positionings of end papers can be used with any combination of the above. Generally, smaller rods will produce smaller, tighter curls and increase the appearance of shortening the hair.

The chemical solution used in the perming process is determined by the client's hair type and the pH of the solution. Classic alkaline perms are used for stronger, coarser hair. They work at room temperature and usually contain ammonium thioglycolate in the pH range of 9-10. Acid perms are used on more delicate or thinner hair. They require outside heat application and usually contain glycerol monothioglycolate in the pH range of 6.5-8.2.

Safety considerations

Due to the harsh nature of the chemicals, it is important that contact with the skin be minimized. Modern chemicals are less irritating, but measures should still be taken to reduce contact with anything other than hair.

A poorly performed permanent wave will result in breakage of the disulfide bonds through chemical reduction, because it fails to fix the newly formed bonds. This results in hair that is no longer elastic and flexible, but brittle and fragile. At this point, even combing the hair will result in hair loss. The hair shafts will experience fracture where they exit the scalp. Because the bulb of hair has not been removed though, the hair follicle is not damaged and the hair will regrow; however, the temporary hair loss may be distressing.

Home perms

A number of brands of home permanent kits are available, but their numbers have decreased as permanent waves are not as popular as they were in the 1980s. The first popular home permanent was the Toni brand. The Toni company used a set of twins to advertise their products — one with a salon perm and one with the home perm. Another brand that was a household name in Britain in the late 1960s and 1970s was Twink.

Reference

(2004). *Salon Fundamentals: A resource for your cosmetology career.* Evanston, IL: Pivot Point International. ISBN 0-6151-1288-9.

External links

- Pictures of Nessler's permanent curling machine
- Disulphide bonds in hair
- The chemistry of a permanent wave
- Old advertisement for Toni brand perm
- Getting a perm in 1950 (demonstration)

The last link shows a permanent-waving demonstration in the United States, in which the 30 apprentices, the demonstrator and the model are all black.

Appendix IV

Eugene v Nessler Patent Trial

The following is a record of a case brought by Eugene against Nestle for infringement of his patent of 1918, which was based on my father's design. The case interesting because it goes into the subtleties of the process, including the use of different temperatures for the root and the end of the hair.

"HISTORY: Appeal from District Court of the United States for the Eastern Division of the Northern District of Ohio; Paul Jones, Judge. Action for infringement of patent by Eugene, Limited, against the Nestle-Le Mur Company. From a decree in favour of plaintiff, defendant appeals. Reversed and remanded, with instructions.

SUMMARY: "Machine" is device or combination of devices by means of which energy can be utilized for useful operation to be performed. Patents for machine, article of manufacture, or composition of matter differ fundamentally in nature from "process" patents. Process may be protected and patented only as a process.

JUDGE: HICKENLOOPER, Circuit Judge Before MOORMAN, HICKS, and HICKENLOOPER, Circuit Judges.

DECISION: 'This is an action for infringement of patent No. 1,266,879, issued to Eugene Francois Suter, May 21, 1918, for electrical heating apparatus for permanently waving hair. Claim 1 is the only claim in suit, and is printed in the margin. The District Court found this claim to be valid and infringed as against defences of anticipation, aggregation, want of invention, and non-infringement. The defendant below appeals. The human hair is waved (permanently, so called) by winding strands or tresses tightly around suitable curlers, dampening with borax solution or other preferred preparation, enclosing these coils in stiff paper tubes, inserting it in tubular electric stoves, and applying heat. The patentee is said to have discovered that, since the hair is coarser and more abundant near the roots, that portion requires heating for a longer period than nearer the tips, where it is finer and more easily injured by excessive heat. To accomplish this result, or practice this method, the patentee duplicated the electric stoves or heaters in common use (see patents to Grosert and Unger, No. 1,103,506, and to Kremer, No. 1,164,102), and connected the electric circuit in parallel to the resistance or heating coils (1), so that by the operation of a switch the current to the upper or outer heater could be connected or disconnected at will. The two heaters are coaxially arranged, attached to each other and held in position by hollow struts through which the electrical connections pass, and except for these struts, are separated by air gaps to prevent heat from passing from one to the other. The method employed by the plaintiff for use of this device is first to connect electrically the lower heater, or that next to the head, and, after that heater has been in operation for a given period of time, to connect the upper or outer heater by means of the switch. Both heaters then remain in use until the waving operation is completed, and thus heat is applied for a longer period to that portion of the hair nearer the roots.

Appendix V

Details of a permanent waving session as described by Bari-Woolls[2]

It seems appropriate to include a contemporary and detailed account of a complete permanent-waving session as carried out in the 1930s. Who better to do this than Bari-Woollss in the conclusion of his book (Ref. 1.). The professional hairdresser may smile at some of the process, not to mention the style, but he may also pick up some interesting or useful information. After detailing a number of competitive processes, he presents the following:

"In this chapter, I propose to run over the practical details of a permanent waving process with my readers using the system with which I am most familiar. This will also serve as a description of a thoroughly up-to-date system which is produced by I. Calvete, Ltd. Mr. I. Calvete is a man whose knowledge of permanent waving machines and their production goes back to 1917 and who has since produced many important inventions in hair-dressing equipment. I will describe a mixed-wound system because I think that this method is bound eventually to become the paramount method of permanent waving.

Our customer enters the cubicle for a permanent wave. After having placed her in the chair and arranged the gown and towels about her we examine the hair, preparatory to shampooing it. If the hair is healthy we proceed with the shampoo in the ordinary way, but if it is badly treated in any way we must consider our technique. First we take the ends of the hair and gently stretch between two fingers. They may stand up to the stretching process well, in which case we may proceed without fear of difficulty because the elasticity retained in that hair will ensure a good perm even if there are several inches of old perm in the ends.

If, on the other hand, the ends break easily we must take special precautions to see that the perm will be successful. Obviously, if the hair is weak and brittle our winding when we come to it will not have to be so tight and our steaming may have to be a little longer. Let us assume then that we have one of those difficult heads to do. Since we are going to steam the hair a little longer than usual we must protect the hair against the power of the extra steam. Thus our shampoo will have to be a little different from an ordinary shampoo. In the case of healthy hair we merely shampoo the hair thoroughly, preferably with a good shampoo of the soapless type which should be neither alkaline nor acid. The hair should be very thoroughly rinsed and then dried completely. This complete drying is essential because any water left in the hair will dilute the reagent and produce a weak perm.

In the case of our weak hair, however, we adopt the special shampoo which is produced for Icall permanent waving known as " Renovex." The hair is shampooed with a soapless shampoo and rinsed, then Renovex is massaged into the hair for five minutes. The hair is then very thoroughly rinsed until all the Renovex is removed and the dryer is placed over the head. When the whole head is dry we begin to taper the hair for the perm.

It is a fact that to obtain the very best results a head of hair should be tapered. This not only takes away the cumbersome weight of the ends, but it aids winding and gives the light curly finish which is so greatly desired these days.

The hair is then ready for winding. If we intended to use the oil process the hair would have to be wetted at this stage with the oil reagent, but as we intend to use sachets and mixed winding a portion of the hair is wound dry. If the ends are badly oversteamed in a previous perm or burnt with Marcel irons a little Renovex can be smeared into the ends as the winding proceeds. A mixed wind is one in which the hair is partly wound on point-wind curlers and partly on root-wind curlers. Since the whole reason for this system of winding is to combine the great strength of curl of point-winding with the perfect waves of root-winding the Icall method recommends that the point-winding be confined to the sides and back of the head where the strength of curl is most required in modern hair fashions. Two rows of point-wind curlers at the sides of the head over the ears and two or three rows at the back of the head according as its size necessitates is usually sufficient to give all the strength and quantity of curl demanded by the most exacting style.

Beginning at the right ear a section of hair is combed just above the ear and on the temple by making a parting running horizontally from the temple. Thus a mesh of hair is taken which is about two and a half inches long by an inch to an inch and a quarter deep. A felt pad of approximately the same size is provided for first protection. It has a slit in the middle of it through which the mesh of hair is drawn. The felt acts as a protector against heat and against any superfluous reagent which might be splashed on the skin. Now the mesh of hair is combed flat and held between the first and second fingers of the right hand. A rubber protector known as a " Presto " Point Protector is taken up open in the left hand with the clip pointing to the right and it is placed so that the flat mesh of hair is between its jaws. This protector is illustrated in Fig. 15. The right hand gently pulls the hair while the left presses the protector close to the scalp. The clip is closed and thus the flat mesh is tightly gripped in a protector in which the grooved edges of the rubber are so closely interlocked that it is impossible for heat or steam to penetrate through to the scalp. It will be noticed that in this protector there is provision for turning the rubber round as it wears in time in order to place a fresh undamaged edge of rubber at the jaws. This, of course, is to give the protector long life.

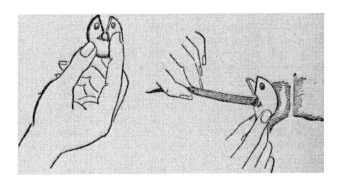

Applying Rubber Protector.

The next mesh of hair of the same size as before is then sectioned or parted off just above the one just protected and another felt and protector placed on that mesh. Using exactly this procedure for each mesh we go on right round the head from the right to the left ear covering the nape of the neck in exactly the same way. It will be found that leaving the top of the head for root winding, the portion of the head just covered requires an average of thirteen or twelve croquignole protectors to cover it. Now, taking into account the size of a mesh of root-wound hair as compared with the mesh used in this type of point winding, there is only half as many curlers used in point winding as would be necessary if the head were wound with this portion done in root winding. This, therefore, is a great saving in time and materials.

Without attempting to wind the point-wound hair at this stage we go straight on to the attaching and winding of the root-wound meshes. The top of the head is as yet untouched. We begin as usual by parting the head off in squares about one inch and a quarter square, commencing at the front of the head over the forehead. The mesh of hair so formed is held in the left hand while the special Icall " Fork " protector, consisting of a flanged, split rubber disc is placed round the roots of the mesh with the right. The rubber disc is then held in the left thumb and finger with the metal studs pointing upwards. The " Fork " Curler is a remarkable invention which allows us to dispense with strings and clips. The curler is held in the right hand and the forked shoe is made to engage by a simple movement with the mesh of hair and the rubber, so that the prongs of the fork are slipped behind the metallic studs. Then the mesh of hair is gently pulled while the rubber protector is pressed down upon the head. Consequently the curler stands erect on the head. It will be found that the rubber so effectively closes the space through which the mesh is pulled that there is no possibility of the head being scalded by escaping steam. Hence when the sachets are put on there will be no need for felt pads, or clips of any description. Of course, if the ordinary two-way curler is used, all that is necessary is that the mesh of hair is pulled through a pierced rubber protector by means of a meshing hook provided and upon which the rubbers are threaded.

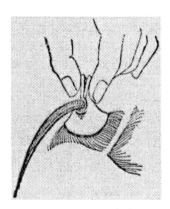 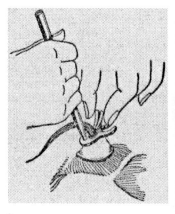

Fixing Curler to Mesh.

Now when this stage is reached the hair is wound on the curler in the way described in previous chapters and the ends held in position with a little teased out crepe hair which is wound in with the ends. Here it is that we decide if the ends are in bad condition to place a little Renovex on them.

We are now ready to put the sachets on these erect curlers. The sachets consist of three pieces of material, first an inner absorbent lint which takes up sufficient reagent to steam the hair, secondly, around that a piece of heat-resistant paper which conserves the steam upon the hair, and finally, surrounding them both a sheet of metal foil which acts as a conductor of heat and by reason of its rigidity when twisted round the curler a means of evenly distributing the heat. It is also a means of attaching them to the curler without the waste of time involved in clipping the older type of sachet upon the mesh with metal or fibre clips. The reagent is supplied in a concentrated form and has to be diluted down for the perm. Since most sachet reagents contain concentrated ammonia we must handle the bottle with care and we must see that it is well stoppered so that the highly volatile ammonia does not escape, so weakening the solution.

The instructions for diluting the reagent are simple and are printed on the label of the bottle, as is usual with most concentrated reagents. If the hair is very impoverished, in this system we use Renovex reagent which is ordinary concentrated reagent which has been diluted down with cold water and Renovex, according to the issued instructions. If the perm were being carried out with any other system we could still use this renovating oil in the reagent or we could use any of the renovating adjuncts to the reagents which their manufacturers supply. There are other emulsion reagents which have a similar effect upon poor hair, such as " Perm-Betta." The reagent having been diluted, the absorbent pads of the sachets are wetted in groups of about a dozen or so and squeezed out so that only sufficient reagent is left in them. They must be damp but not running wet. Thus by pressing them well between a folded towel this condition of even dampness can be easily brought about. The damp sachets with their paper and metal foil are then wrapped around the curlers and nothing more has to be done to them beyond the steaming.

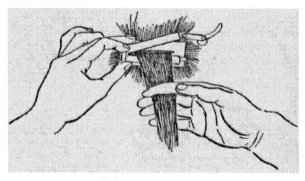

Applying Presto Protector.

We are now ready for point-winding. The hair which is hanging from the point-wind or Presto protectors is wetted with reagent, the same reagent as is used for the rest of the hair, and we begin to wind. The Presto curler is a metal spool with no clip on it to make a frizzy clip-mark but with just a series of serrations in the middle which grip the points of the hair.

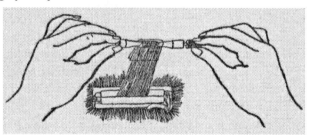

Winding Presto Curler.

The hair is combed flat and the ends are caught up in a strip of thin folded cellophane which keeps the points flat while enabling the operator to see whether he is winding them properly. Thus the cellophane and hair are wound together from the points

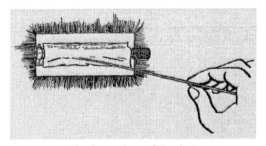

Closing edge of Sachet.

keeping the mesh as tight and as flat as possible. It is recommended that in wetting the mesh with reagent the three quarters of an inch close to the protector be left dry since that will be covered with a sachet. The hair is wound over the top of the curler and if any stray tapered ends tend to fall down they are wound in with the aid of a thin steel winding needle. Upon winding close up to the protector the hexagonal nut at the left end of the curler fits into a hexagonal slot in the protector while the head of the curler fits into its the slot at the right end of the protector. Just as the Fork curler is a one-way self-tightening curler so is the Presto curler. A mere turn of the right end; there is a slot by which a coin enables extreme tightness to be obtained; and the curler is tightened to the fullest extent.

The Presto sachets are then damped with reagent in the same way as the "Fork" sachets and are pressed into position over the curlers. The metal foil of the sachet is worked with the end of the needle so that it fits very closely to the hair and the whole head is ready for steaming.

Had we intended to use the " Icall-H " machine a different reagent suitable for falling-heat permanent waving would have been used and the machine which had been switched on previously would now be alternating between its display of red and white lights. This machine would only be put to the curlers when the light was showing red, but in the perm we are describing now we intend to use the "Icall " COMBINATION MACHINE.

The head ready for steaming appears as in the illustration on page

The machine is drawn up to the head with the standard in line with the nape of the neck and the crown about two feet above the top of the head. The " Safex " Heaters are put over the root-wound hair and the Presto Heaters are clipped over the point-wound meshes. The Safex Heater is one in which every source of danger in permanent waving has been remedied as far as is possible with direct electrical heating. The element is encased hermetically in a metal covering which prevents either reagent or air from entering and corroding the electrical wiring. The connecting leads are placed in separate chambers made of a unique synthetic resin which will not succumb to very high temperatures. The whole heater is surrounded by a case of the same material which so completely keeps the outside of the heater cool that there is no fear of discomfort even if it is handled when at full heat. The makers claim that because of its massive external earthing connection which effectively earths every portion of the heater which might come into contact with undesired electrical currents it is the only permanent waving heater which strictly follows the ruling of the Institute of Electrical Engineers in the matter of earthing.

The Presto Heaters are designed to obtain the same quality of safety combined with the most efficient heating of the whole mesh of hair that is possible. By close application to the consequences of such design the makers have been able to produce a mixed-wind system in which the steaming time is the same for both classes of winding.

When the heaters are placed in position the current is switched on and the heaters begin to do their work. The heaters are produced to steam the hair uniformly over the whole head and to that end it takes exactly four minutes for the mesh to reach the steaming point. Therefore, we do not have to bother about watching the colour of the sachets or waiting for steam to be visible at their ends. The machine is equipped with standard uniform heaters upon which we can completely rely.

But the vagaries of the electrical supply are outside of our control; in the mornings when there is a great demand for power the voltage of the electrical supplies may be low, while during the evenings when most people go over to more economical lighting currents the voltage will rise considerably. Again the wiring of the saloon may be poor, with the result that the voltage may not be as high as we think. Without exact knowledge of the voltage our permanent wave may be a failure.

If the voltage is too high the machine will steam more quickly and the perm will be too tight. This may render it almost impossible to produce a good rewave when the customer returns to us in six months time. To obviate the dangers of such fluctuations of voltage the Icall Machine is fitted with an Auto-Timing Switch. This splendid aid to the hairdresser is a combined high precision voltmeter and an automatic self-winding clock. As soon as the current is switched on the voltmeter tells us the exact voltage of the supply upon which we are working and immediately informs us whether there is a rise above or a fall below the rating of the heaters. If the voltage is too high it will necessitate a reduction of steaming time while if low it will be essential to increase the steaming time. Engraved on the case of the auto-timing switch are the correct instructions whereby exact modifications of the steaming time can be made to suit the various conditions. Thus this useful mechanism eliminates guesswork from our steaming and throws the only onus upon our knowledge of the condition and texture of the hair to be waved. The automatic clock is set for the corrected time (corrected for voltage as the voltmeter indicates) and at that time a warning *buzzer* reminds us that it is time to remove the heaters. When this time arrives the heaters are switched off and removed.

On no account must the hair be taken off the curlers until they are quite cool but the sachets may be removed immediately and indeed should be in order to facilitate this cooling. At this stage the Fork curlers are then removed by a simple twist of the hair in the reverse direction to the wind and the point-wound curlers are simply pressed to the left when they will come off just as easily. The hair will, if it has been correctly steamed, be found to be still damp. It is combed out to render the shampoo and setting easier, it is then shampooed, put in pli, dried and dressed out. No matter what style of dressing is required it is simple to obtain it with this type of process.

The Icall Machine may be adapted by the addition of simple metallic rings in the mouth of the heater and centralising caps on the top into perfect oil heaters so that it is truly an universal heater which will enable us to produce oil perms with any reputable oil reagent and sachet perms with any efficient sachet. Carried out in the way described and with the logical understanding of the theory of permanent waving which I have endeavoured to place upon paper in this little work, success in the art of the permanent waver is assured. The speed of the system which has just been described is phenomenal, for without great trouble an average time of one hour and a half for perming, shampooing, setting and dressing out, can be easily attained with the Icall COMBINATION SYSTEM."

Appendix VI

The Deptford Power Stations[13]

This Appendix has been extracted from the website www.swehs.co, produced by the South Western Electricity Historical Society (Histelec News No. 25) with their kind permission, as I believe it relevant to the development of power stations in London and hence to the power required for all applications electrical equipment, including hairdressing. The original is a pamphlet published by the CEGB in 1986 entitled "Cradle of Power – The Story of Deptford Power Stations" and written by Rob Cochrane. The pamphlet came to light, when historical material was rescued from The Electricity Association's offices at Millbank before being closed down.

"Deptford was to see the start of a development, which would make possible so many of the technological achievements of the 20th Century through the large-scale generation of electricity and its high voltage transmission over great distances inaugurated in the Deptford power station scheme. It's difficult to realise fully the immensity of the step forward at that time, and to appreciate the vision of the man responsible - Sebastian de Ferranti - not to mention his courage in confronting the beliefs of eminent men of science. The industrial revolution had transformed manufacturing processes, transport was horse-drawn and the motor car was only just being invented. For most people, lighting was provided by candles or paraffin lamps. Although the use of gas was increasing in towns, the 'bats-wing' burners gave only a poor light.

Electric lighting was in its infancy. Michael Faraday's discovery of electro-magnetic induction in 1831 had opened the way to converting mechanical power into electricity, and within thirty years small generators were being used in lighthouses. By 1878 the Sheffield Football Association had staged an evening match under electric lights - with players' errors being blamed on the intensity of the illumination. The Gaiety Theatre was using some electric lighting, and the next year saw the start of the famous Blackpool illuminations. But until that time lighting had been produced by the arcing of electricity between two carbon rods, with an intensity and glare, which made it quite unsuitable for normal domestic use. The effect of the electric lighting at the Gaiety had been described as 'half a dozen harvest moons shining at once in the Strand', while a committee appointed by a gas company reassured shareholders by reporting 'We are quite satisfied that the electric light can never be applied indoors without the production of an offensive smell, which undoubtedly causes headaches, and in its naked state it can never be used in rooms of even a large size without damage to sight'.

The breakthrough came with Joseph Swan's invention of the incandescent lamp, matched in the United States by an almost simultaneous invention by Thomas Edison. An installation in the new Savoy Theatre, opened in 1880 by Richard D'Oyly Carte for the Gilbert and Sullivan Operas, was claimed by that impresario to be 'the first time it has been attempted to light any public building entirely by electricity'. A year later the House of Commons was similarly lit, but electric lighting was still something of a status symbol for businesses and individuals, with small experimental local stations being set up in the West End and the wealthier residential districts.

It was in 1883 that Sir Coutts Lindsay made up his mind to light his Grosvenor Gallery in New Bond Street with 'the new smokeless electricity'. A neighbour to whom he mentioned the idea promptly said 'Put down twice the necessary machinery and produce twice the current you need, and let me have what you can spare'. Soon others were making similar requests and the original installation in an outbuilding became quite inadequate to meet all requirements. Sir Coutts decided to build a permanent generating station in a specially constructed basement under the Gallery. Three steam engines drove a pair of Siemens alternators - the largest yet built by that pioneer electrical company - the current being transmitted to other premises by overhead cables supported from poles on the housetops. However, the system installed at that time proved so difficult to work that he invited a 21-year-old engineer named Ferranti to take charge of the generating station: a step which was to have momentous consequences.

Man of Vision

Sebastian Ziani de Ferranti was already a remarkable young man ; not altogether surprising considering the family from which he came. Two of his ancestors had been elected Doges of Venice during the 12th Century, and later members of his family had held important positions in the Italian city states of the Middle Ages. His grandfather was a musician of distinction - a friend of Paganini and Rossini. His father had become famous as a portrait photographer, while his mother was a highly accomplished musician who, until the death of her first husband, had toured all the European capitals with him giving recitals. Yet from a very early age, Sebastian's whole interest was focused on engineering and scientific matters.

When he entered St Augustine's Roman Catholic College at Ramsgate, he was lucky in having as headmaster a man of great insight. Sebastian's schoolwork showed anything but promise, yet Abbot Regan recognised his developing qualities. 'That he was an original genius soon became perceptible... he forced us to let him have full scope for his ingenuity, and we willingly assigned him a room, where all by himself, he could work at practical problems, exercising his budding genius.'

Within a month of leaving St Augustine's at seventeen, he had sold a dynamo he had made for £5 10s 0d and soon got employment with Siemens, being sent around the country to supervise the installation of electric lighting plants. By eighteen he had set up his own company in collaboration with Alfred Thompson, an engineer, and Francis Ince, a lawyer greatly interested in scientific developments; and that same year of 1882 saw another remarkable achievement. He invented an alternator with a revolutionary type of zig-zag armature, which far outstripped anything else on the market at that time; only to find that another machine with many identical features had just been developed by Sir William Thomson (later Lord Kelvin). Agreement was reached under which the machine marketed was known as the Thomson-Ferranti alternator, with Sir William receiving a royalty on all sales.

That early achievement was impressive enough in the light of developments in this country, where the use of electricity was lagging far behind the United States and some European countries. Here the industry was little more than a collection of huts and basements with clanking reciprocating steam engines supplying lamps within a relatively small radius. Even a 'big' station would generate no more than 800 kilowatts - enough to light 26,000 lamps of that period; but the level of illumination they gave was poor, and the most that could be said was that it was better than anything else then available. But already a major challenge was on its way.

In 1886 Welsbach had invented the incandescent gas mantle, increasing the efficiency of gas lighting. Gas had already been a much cheaper means of lighting than electricity, and was being made even more economic by gas companies shutting down local gasworks in favour of much bigger plants situated in places like Rotherhithe.

208

The Grand Design

Ferranti didn't hesitate to use the gas industry's example in support of his own vision. In place of a proliferation of little electric light works serving local communities he envisaged a big power station capable of supplying London with electricity on a really large scale, built by the Thames where unlimited cooling water was available and where land and the seaborne supplies of coal would be cheap. 'The business of distributing electrical energy must be done on a large scale to be commercial, and to attain this we must supply a large area ... and we must do this from a site not in the congested heart of a big city but from a position best suited by its natural advantages to the carrying on of such an undertaking.'

The scheme he planned was on a scale undreamed of in this or any other country. It says much for the acumen and financial courage of Sir Coutts Lindsay and his brother Lord Wantage that they formed and were the principal shareholders of the London Electric Supply Corporation Ltd having anauthorised capital of £1,000,000, with the intention that LESCo should take over the Grosvenor Gallery station and proceed with the massive new undertaking. And it was decided to build this new station at Deptford on a 3-acre site called The Stowage, which had once housed the store rooms, rigging sheds, mast sheds and sail lofts of the East India Company.

It was an incredible venture for its time. The plant at the Gallery was already considered big, but Ferranti's proposals must have seemed like a leap into the technical unknown. Whereas the largest of the four Gallery engines was 750 hp, the Deptford plant would eventually include four of 10,000 hp each. Instead of the existing four boilers capable of producing 20,000 lbs of steam per hour, the new station would have eighty boilers with a steaming capacity of 1,380,000 lbs per hour - and it was planned to triple even that arrangement. But perhaps the most startling aspect was the proposal to install at Deptford four alternators of 500 tons each, generating at 10,000 volts and more than twelve times the capacity of the Grosvenor Gallery alternators. The completed station would be capable of supplying no less than two million lamps.

Work began in April 1888, and was pushed forward night and day to such effect that by midsummer 1889 the main building had been erected, 24 boilers and two initial 1,250 hp engines had been installed and the alternators were almost ready. Ferranti's part in this almost beggars description. His wife wrote later, 'The first thing I remembered during those first months of married life was Deptford, and again Deptford. We talked Deptford and dreamed Deptford'. On many nights he didn't go to bed at all, staying in a little cottage on site which he used as an office and sometimes spreading his overcoat on the floor and lying down to snatch an hour or two's sleep. The Chairman of LESCo was generous in his praise:' He pledged his reputation, his fortune, his labour - day and night - to achieve the result he promised to the Directors'.

There was no aspect in which he wasn't personally involved. In October 1888 the Electrical Engineer quoted him as "The Michelangelo of that installation because from first to last, from foundation to highest turret, the architecture, materials, foundations and machines all were specified or designed by one man, and the credit of that success will have to be given, without detracting one iota in favour of any other person, to Ferranti".

He wasn't without his critics. Eminent men of the day prophesied disaster, particularly in Ferranti's proposed use of the unheard of electrical pressure of 10,000 volts to transmit the current to central London. That pressure seems very ordinary nowadays, when the British Supergrid operates at 400,000 volts, but at the time it created a sensation. As one writer put it, anything over 2,000 volts was regarded as dangerous and tempting Providence. The heart of the matter was the belief held by many very distinguished engineers that the future of electricity supply lay in direct current low-tension systems, serving local communities. Ferranti was convinced that economic electricity supply depended on the use of alternating current and transformers, which would enable the energy to be transmitted at high voltage over very much greater distances. The 'Battle of the Systems' - AC versus DC - was to rage for years. One of the exponents of the DC system was Thomas Edison, hailed by many as the genius of the age. Even before Sir Coutts Lindsay had started his Grosvenor Gallery station, two of Edison's renowned 'Jumbo Dynamos' (named after a circus elephant) had been installed in the 3,000 light generating station at No.57 Holborn Viaduct; the first central station for private incandescent lighting in the world, which came into operation in January 1882, just a few months before Edison's own famous Pearl Street station in New York. In September 1889 the famous man visited the Deptford power station under construction.

The Daily News told how, despite his severe cold, he 'soon appeared to forget his indisposition when he began his inspection of the wonderful machinery, spending a long time minutely examining the immense engines and dynamos'. With his convictions about the immense superiority of low tension systems he was hardly an unbiased observer, and spoke of the risks of an enormous electrical pressure through a narrow wire compared with 'our New York tension wires which are so safe that even a child may play with them'. But he added 'Oh, it will go!' Others abroad were following the progress of the Deptford Station with great interest. The New York Electrical World admitted combined admiration and apprehension about the proposed high tension method of transmission - the project must be either a gigantic success or gigantic failure - but it was unstinting in its appreciation of the concept:

"The reproach which has long existed regarding the backward state of electric lighting in England is at last to be removed. ... There is now in progress in London an installation which is calculated to exceed many times in capacity any other existing light installation in the world .etc".

For Ferranti to envisage transmitting current at such a high pressure was one thing; to achieve it proved quite a different matter. The cables originally purchased and laid in the early part of 1889 were a failure. He decided that the only way to get mains capable of transmitting current at 10,000 volts to central London would be to design and manufacture his own; the beginning of the famous Ferranti cables, and another achievement generously applauded in the public press.

Within six months, the London Daily News was carrying a story: 'The Ferranti "mains" are believed to be one of the most valuable discoveries yet made in electric lighting. The "main" or cable contains, within the same casing, both the conductor for the "out" current and the conductor for the "return" current; and it may be laid down in the earth without any protection whatever. It consists of two copper tubes, one within the other, separated by an insulating substance; outside the outer tube is another layer of the insulating substance (Mr. Ferranti's invention) and the whole is inserted into a protecting tube of iron. The "mains" thus completed are laid down in lengths of twenty feet each. They now extend from Deptford, through Charing Cross to the distributing station at Maiden Lane. This is the section which will be ready to supply some twenty thousand glow lamps of ten candle power each on the 1st October.' (Ferranti's 'insulating substance' consisted of layers of chemically pure brown paper, saturated with melted earthwax; the 'protecting tube of iron' was added after the initial design.)

That newspaper may have told the story: but it didn't recount the whole story! The power company knew that the cable-laying would involve having to break up some streets, involving all the delays and expense of obtaining statutory powers. To reduce the need for this, agreement was reached with three railway companies by which the mains were to be laid on the surface along railway tracks and across the bridges to the Charing Cross, Cannon Street and Blackfriars stations. A similar agreement with the Metropolitan and District Underground Railway enabled their tunnels to be used to get the cables to the main distribution points.

That was all very well: but the Board of Trade, responsible for ensuring the public safety of electricity supply, was more than sceptical whether Ferranti had provided an effective means of earthing a 10,000 volt current in the event of mishap. He promptly invited them to witness a highly unusual demonstration. Harold Kolle, who had left his previous post of Electrical Engineer at Eastbourne to join him, volunteered to hold a cold chisel while another assistant drove it through a live main! Both remained completely unscathed. But even though permission to proceed was given, the job of cable laying had its more interesting moments.

At first, the junction between each of the 20 ft cable lengths had been filled with black wax forced in under pressure: until a pump burst and splattered a newly varnished shop-front with wax, and a new jointing method had to be hastily devised. Then there was the time when a navvies foreman decided that a cast-iron pipe they had uncovered must be one of the many London street pipes no longer in use: until they cut into it and a huge jet of water shot high over the neighbouring roofs. Sacks of stones and wheelbarrows hastily piled on top did no good at all, and the deluge continued until an official hastily summoned from the water company could find the valve and turn if off. 'There was a terrible mess - - - - and the most terrible row!'

Yet in spite of everything the cables were laid, and out of 8,000 joints only 15 proved faulty. It was an impressive achievement. Some of those cables were to remain in regular service until 1933, only being replaced then because of the need to provide greater compatibility in the cable system. Under the heading 'Sic Transit! End of the Famous 10,000 volt Ferranti Cables of Glorious Memory' the Electrical Times commemorated the fortyfive years' history of 'the first paper-insulated concentrics ever made, and the forerunners of those that we know today'. As they said, 'It is a wonderful record'.

Disappointment and Disaster

Yet even while Ferranti had been working on the design of the high voltage cables, a massive blow had been dealt to his plans for a really effective and economical supply of electricity to London from the Deptford station; and ironically, this arose from the commonplace need to lay the low voltage distribution cables in the streets.

LESCo had made a wholesale application for the necessary statutory authority covering streets within the boundaries of 24 local authorities; something quite unprecedented in sheer scale for laying electricity cables, which happened to coincide with a number of smaller applications from other companies. The Board of Trade promptly ordered a local enquiry. For them, this was an opportunity to regulate a whole sphere of operations of electricity supply undertakings by laying down principles under which powers to break up streets would be granted - as well as a chance of examining the whole scope of the revolutionary Deptford proposals.

To Ferranti, the effects of the inquiry under Major Marindin were nothing less than catastrophic. Under pressure of the argument that the concentration of four 10,000 hp units at Deptford would constitute a risk of maintaining a reliable electricity supply, the LESCo Directors agreed to put two of the units in a station to be built elsewhere. Worse, Deptford's proposed area of supply was halved. And, in the area still left, Ferranti could foresee the likely effect of the general principle adopted as a result of the inquiry: that while a local authority might allow two companies to compete within its area, they should not both supply alternating current, a measure tacitly encouraging the further growth of local low-tension stations. As he explained in a letter written some years later:

"Failure to maintain our position at the Government inquiry entirely killed the scheme. Our area was greatly reduced, but worse than this, we had competition from local stations arranged for in every part of our area ... naturally with a new system on the scale we were operating, it was very difficult to compete right away with the small low-tension stations dotted

213

all over our area as, of course, we had great technical difficulties to deal with at the start, and the small low-tension stations had very little new to contend with".

That was still for the future. At the time, in spite of his feelings about the result of the inquiry, Ferranti was keeping up the pressure to bring the station into operation. By November 1889 the first generating unit was brought into service; and although this was only a 1,250 hp machine, it was more than capable of providing all the electricity supplies that would be required until the original mains cables could be replaced by the 10,000 volt cables he had designed. A few months later he was reporting that two of the 10,000 hp engines had been completed in manufacturer's works, the 10,000 volt alternators were in an advanced state and soon the whole of that major generating capacity would be at the company's disposal.

Even those plans were never to be realised, destroyed as the result of one man's simple error. It happened on 15th November 1890, while the engine room machinery at the Grosvenor Gallery was being dismantled and the electricity supply to customers was being provided by incoming supplies from Deptford. An operator at the Gallery was bringing a fresh set of transformers into service when he mishandled a switch and started a 5,000 volt electrical arc. He must have momentarily lost his head; instead of cutting off the current, he allowed the arc to continue, starting a fire which swept through the whole of the station. It was a major setback, doubly unfortunate because the extent of the damage was due to a temporary rearrangement of plant while Deptford was taking over responsibility for generation; but worse was to follow.

Everyone rose to the occasion. By a superhuman effort, supplies to customers were restored within a fortnight by repairing some of the less badly damaged transformers and getting hold of some new ones. Then only a week later one of the repaired transformers failed, throwing its electrical load onto the others; and as they were already carrying as much current as they could safely, they burned out one after the other. As the Directors weren't confident that the Deptford station was really ready to carry the full load, they decided to cease all attempts to give any supply until this could be done reliably.

The shutdown lasted three months, and none of that time was wasted. The overhead lines from the Grosvenor Gallery were replaced with 24 cables, while at the same time the 10,000 volt cables from Deptford to central London were completed. But by then the damage was done. Many customers had deserted the company, and the number of lamps connected to the system had dwindled from 38,000 to 9,000. It's not surprising that the LESCo Directors were worried men, finding it difficult to maintain faith in Ferranti's bold concept. The company had lost a lot of money. The hopes of achieving large scale supplies of electricity to London seemed to be vanishing before their eyes, while many of the most eminent men in the field were still insisting that the future of electricity lay with much smaller low-tension stations.

Ferranti had his supporters of his scheme, which history would eventually prove right. It was quite another matter for the Company's Directors in that May of 1891. They could see that the two 400 kilowatt alternators transferred to Deptford from the Grosvenor Gallery were more than sufficient to meet all requirements at that time: and soon the two original 1,250 hp units would be back in service after their alternators had been rewound to raise their voltage to 10,000 volts. What need for the immense 10,000 hp machines originally planned and awaiting installation? The wrath of LESCo Chairman J S Forbes descended on the young engineer: 'Ye're a very clever man, Mr. Ferranti, but I'm thinking ye're sadly lacking in prevision'. The order for the machines was cancelled. For Ferranti, that must have spelt the end of his vision of Deptford as a station capable of meeting much of London's increasing demand for electricity with the economic benefits of large scale generation. As he was to comment later, 'Not long after these events occurred, all the in-town stations were in such trouble from one cause or another that they were looking for supply from outside. If Deptford had been continued on its right lines, it would have been able to furnish current wholesale for distribution by other companies.' As it was, he left the Company in the August of 1891 to resume his manufacturing career.

However even with Ferranti gone, Deptford was back in service by August 1891. The Company's old customers were returning as fast as they could be reconnected. But by November of that year, the system had collapsed again. They soldiered on for a few more years until in 1900, it was decided to shutdown for 6 months in order to replace both cables and plant. From then on the Deptford Station went from strength to strength, culminating in a further power station being built alongside, called "Deptford West" and being commissioned in 1929. Deptford East as the old station became known was rejuvenated in 1953 when an extension was built to accommodate an HP station, known as Deptford East HP. Generation ceased on site finally in 1983."

Appendix VII

Economic Indices for the Inter-War Period

It is always difficult making comparisons of prices after the passage of considerable time. The following table[2] gives the changes in the value of the pound during the period discussed in this book and the present, taking the 1920 value to be 100.

	1920	1930	1939	2004
Retail Price Index (RPI)	100	63	64	4095
Gross Domestic Product (GDP)	100	67	70	4465
Individual Earnings	100	70	99	16510

The retail price index or RPI is the simplest measure of inflation measured from the price of a basket of standard consumer items. While today the cost of living increases continuously to a lesser or greater degree due to inflation, after 1920 the RPI went down, that is, inflation was negative, things got cheaper (but earnings lessened), until 1923 and then levelled off until the War. As the 2004 index is about 41 times the 1930 index, this factor has been used to give an idea of the cost of some items.

The Gross Domestic Product started going down after the First World War and settled in 1922 remaining fairly constant until 1936, but dropped suddenly in 1939 with the prospect of war.

Unemployment was high during the interwar period, reaching a peak in 1932 of 22.1%.

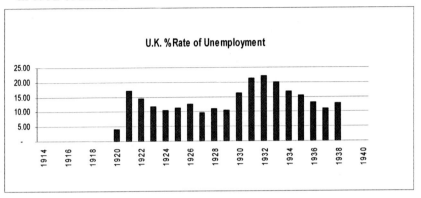

On the whole, this twenty-year period gives a picture of industrial, economic and political instability, not aided by the Great Strike, the Wall Street Crash of 1929 and subsequent strikes in Britain. In fact, the period was characterised by massive unemployment both in the United Kingdom and abroad, made worse by inadequate unemployment benefits.

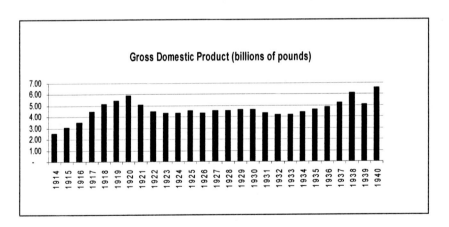

Appendix VIII

Obituary of Karl Nessler

In February 1951, the Hairdressers' Journal published an obituary on Karl Nessler giving him the attention he did not receive during his first publicised permanent-waving session. The details seem to have come largely from the United States where he died and so have an American slant. I would query some of the statements when compared with those from other sources, so I have added some footnotes to deal with these.

DEATH OF CHARLES NESSLER[a]

It is with deep regret that we announce the death of Mr. Charles Nessler who originated the permanent waving-process. He died on January 22 at his home in Harrington Park, New Jersey, U.S.A. He had been unwell for some time, and the cause of death was a heart attack. He was 78.

Mr. Nessler, a Swiss[2], became a barber-surgeon in his native country. In 1905, he gave his first lecture on the theory of hair-waving. His claims evoked such widespread interest that he began experimenting with a machine which he could use in his demonstrations. This task occupied about four years.. He left Switzerland and opened a salon in London, where he launched his permanent waving device.

In the suceeding years, he operated various West End Salons with enormous success. At these salons, permanent waving for the public, on a commercial basis, was established as a routine cubicle operation before 1910. One of his highly successful salons was at 48, South Molton Street.

There is no dispute among craft historians that Mr. Nessler gave chemical permanent waving to the Trade; it is not so certain, however, whether he should be given the sole credit for inventing the electrical heater, which came later.[3]

With the long hair styles then fashionable, and only two heaters on the machine, a permanent wave would take most of the day. Later, Nessler devised various systems for allowing other hairdressers to use his invention; one was for an initial licensing payment of £30, plus 4s. for each curler applied to a customer.[4]

Soon after the start of the First World War, Mr. Nessler decided to leave England. He arrived in America in 1915 and opened a shop on East Fort-Sixth Street, under the name of Nestlé. Among his first customers was Mrs Woodrow Wilson, wife of the U.S. President. As a result of her patronage, Mr. Nessler's success was immediate and before long he was charging $120 (about £30) for a wave.

A great showman and a lovable character, he was known by his staff as Father Nestlé. All his patrons were served with a free lunch. His success inspired intensive competition and he was frequently obliged to indulge in litigation to protect his interests. One of the companies which he sued for patent infringement was a Cleveland concern to which, in 1928, he sold his corporation. It became known as the Nestlé-Le-Mur Company.

Mr. Nessler's theory was based on the tendency of damp hair to curl. His device was intended to make hair porous enough to absorb moisture after which he processed it with heat and an alkaline solution to preserve the curl. His methods and theories formed the subject of his book, *The Story of Hair*.

Many organisations throughout America honoured him in recent years with special citations and awards, including the Women's Voluntary Association which in 1949 feted him for having enhanced the beauty of women and given them opportunities in the beauty trade. Hollywood should also be grateful to him, for it was he who invented false eyelashes.[5]

Charles Nessler will always be remembered as the founder of a major industry and as a man who put friendship before gain.

My Notes:

1. He was originally Karl Nessler, but he seems to have anglicised his forename in America. He used the name Nestlé for business purposes.

2. All his earlier references give him as German, which tallies with his escape from Britain at the First World War to avoid internment. Switzerland was not a combatant nation.

3. The underlining is mine. The central thesis of this book is that practical permanent waving using appropriately designed electrical heaters did not take place until the meeting and collaboration of Calvete and Eugene in 1917.

4. The very high cost and time taken for the process, plus the use of harsh reagents on the hair, show that the Nessler process as it stood originally could never become the popular process it would was to become. On the other hand, Nessler was perhaps the earliest to combine the principle of heat (as in Marcel-waving), moisture in the form of steam and some alkaline chemical to assist in altering the structure of the hair.

5. This may not be the place to start on the history of false eyelashes (or finger-nails) but any student of the subject should read Reference 24, which shows how the brothers Aylott originated the business and supplied many of the famous stars of both Hollywood and Britain with a business which they started up in 1946, in Welwyn Garden City, England.

Appendix IX

London's West End – Location of Relevant Sites

The map on the next page shows how many of the early events in this book took place in the West End of London. – in the elegant salons of Mayfair and in the workshops of Soho.

Although, naturally, permanent-waving and its adjuncts spread all over the world, it is interesting that in the United Kingdom at least it seems to have largely originated in a quite small area of London, the styles in elegant Mayfair and the first factories in less-exalted Soho. When in full swing, Eugene moved its supply activities northwards to Hendon and I. Calvete Ltdits manufacturing southwards to Clapham. This is not to diminish the contributions made by other manufacturers, including those from other countries. France, and its stylists in Paris, and Germany were particularly important.

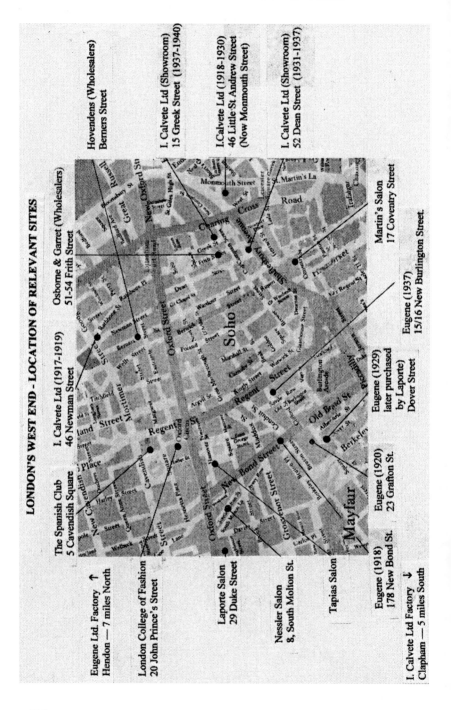

LONDON'S WEST END - LOCATION OF RELEVANT SITES

Hovendens (Wholesalers)
Berners Street

I. Calvete Ltd (Showroom)
15 Greek Street (1937-1940)

I.Calvete Ltd (1918-1930)
46 Little St Andrew Street
(Now Monmouth Street)

I. Calvete Ltd (Showroom) (1931-1937)
52 Dean Street

Martin's Salon
17 Coventry Street

Eugene (1937)
15/16 New Burlington Street

Eugene (1929)
later purchased
by Laporte)
Dover Street

Eugene (1920)
23 Grafton St.

Eugene (1918)
178 New Bond St.

I. Calvete Ltd Factory
Clapham — 5 miles South

Tapias Salon

Nessler Salon
8, South Molton St.

Laporte Salon
29 Duke Street

London College of Fashion
20 John Prince's Street

Eugene Ltd Factory
Hendon — 7 miles North

The Spanish Club
5 Cavendish Square

I. Calvete Ltd (1917-1919)
46 Newman Street

Osborne & Garret (Wholesalers)
51-54 Frith Street

Glossary

Chandelier   The circular upper support of a permanent machine which took the weight of the heaters and also distributed electricity to them.

Croquignole   See point winding.

Heater   A device for heating the hair either directly or more properly by creating steam. In most cases, heating was carried out, either directly or indirectly, by electricity.

Méche   Lock of hair

Point winding.   Winding the hair on to the curler starting from the ends of the hair. Also called croquignole.

Reagent: Generally an aqueous solution of certain chemicals, such as borax, ammonia, etc. which enhances the waving process.

Root winding   Winding the hair on to the curler starting from the roots of the hair.

Sachet   A pad with an impermeable membrane, which was wetted and then wrapped around the hair-winding before steaming.

Steaming   Heating the hair with steam, rather than by dry heat. Steam transfers the heat more efficiently and at the same time softens the hair making waving easier.

Some contemporary exhibitions of equipment and hairdressing competitions

1925   Wembley - Ideal Home Exhibition
1926   October. Exhibition
1927   Beauty Exhibition, Holland Park
          British Industries Federation Exhibition
1928   British Industries Federation Exhibition
1929   Hairdressing Fair of Fashion and Beauty
1930   Frankfurt Exhibition Germany
          British Industries Federation Exhibition
          Hairdressers' Exhibition Olympia
          Daily Mail Ideal Home Exhibition March/April
1931   Buenos Aires Exhibition
          Hairdressers' Exhibition, Paris
1932   British Industries Federation Exhibition, Olympia (March)
1934   British Industries Federation Exhibition, Birmingham
1935   British Industries Fed. Exhibition, Agricultural Hall London.
1936   Hair and Beauty Fair, Olympia (October)
1938   Hair and Beauty Fair, Olympia (September)

INDEX

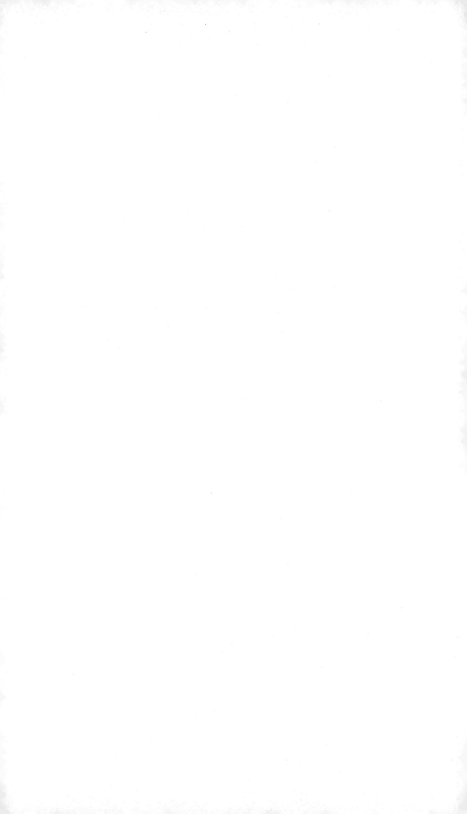

Printed in the United Kingdom
by Lightning Source UK Ltd.
117720UKS00001B/109-117